Robert P. Langlais, B.A., D.D.S., M.S.
Professor, Department of Dental Diagnostic Science
University of Texas Health Science Center Dental School
San Antonio, Texas

Myron J. Kasle, D.D.S., M.S.D.
Professor and Chairman, Department of Dental Radiology
Indiana University School of Dentistry
Indianapolis, Indiana

EXERCISES IN
Oral Radiographic Interpretation

SECOND EDITION

1985

W. B. Saunders Company
Philadelphia London Toronto
Mexico City Rio de Janeiro Sydney Tokyo

W. B. Saunders Company: West Washington Square
Philadelphia, PA   19105

1 St. Anne's Road
Eastbourne, East Sussex BN21 3UN, England

1 Goldthorne Avenue
Toronto, Ontario M8Z 5T9, Canada

Apartado 26370—Cedro 512
Mexico 4, D.F., Mexico

Rua Coronel Cabrita, 8
Sao Cristovao Caixa Postal 21176
Rio de Janeiro, Brazil

9 Waltham Street
Artarmon, N.S.W. 2064, Australia

Ichibancho, Central Bldg., 22-1 Ichibancho
Chiyoda-Ku, Tokyo 102, Japan

Listed here are the latest translated editions of this book together with the language of the translation and the publisher.

German (1st Edition)—Georg Thieme Verlag, Stuttgart, Germany

Italian (1st Edition)—Editrice Cides Odonto Edizioni Internazionali, Torino, Italy

Spanish (1st Edition)—El Manual Moderno S.A., Mexico City, Mexico

Library of Congress Cataloging in Publication Data

Langlais, Robert P.

Exercises in oral radiographic interpretation.

Rev. ed. of: Intra-oral radiographic interpretation. 1978.

Includes index.

1. Teeth—Radiography—Problems, exercises, etc.   I. Kasle, Myron J.   II. Langlais, Robert P. Intra-oral radiographic interpretation.   III. Title. [DNLM: 1. Radiography, Dental—examination questions. WN 18 L282i]

RK309.L34 1985   617.6'07572'076   84–29832

ISBN 0–7216–1497–3

Exercises in Oral Radiographic Interpretation   ISBN   0–7216–1497–3

Last digit is the print number: 9   8   7   6   5   4   3   2   1

To our teachers—our students

Foreword
to the First Edition

Dental radiology is the "Cinderella" of dentistry, and despite the fact that it is well taught in most dental schools, it is on the whole poorly learned by the average practicing dentist, although there are many who have substantial or even great interest in its pursuit. The quality of dental radiographic technique is, in general, equally poor, so that as a consequence, most dentists are unacquainted with the radiographic appearances of all but a few of the most common pathological processes that may occur in and about the teeth and jaws. As a rare consequence of this, serious or even grave outcomes occur for the patients.

Dental schools differ in their attitudes toward the value of radiology in dental education and practice, and some schools have no oral radiologist. This is detrimental not only to the education of the student but also to the standard of radiologic service within the institution, perhaps most noticeably in the department of surgery where maximal help is needed but is often not forthcoming.

Good textbooks exist, but readers have to be motivated to read them, and adequate motivation is often lacking once the student has graduated and entered practice. Most of these textbooks use a didactic approach, but this one of Drs. Langlais and Kasle is somewhat Socratic and is also highly imaginative, for alongside the many illustrations that have been selected for their pertinent contents, searching questions are asked that are designed to engender interest, to instruct, and to exercise the mind. As a similar format is used in examinations, students are indoctrinated to become familiar with this method. Answers are supplied that illuminate the information inherent in the selected radiographic illustrations. Imagination has been used in selecting appropriate illustrations and sensitive prescience in posing searching questions directed to educating the observer and student. Thus, student and practitioner can, if they wish, increase their knowledge of interpretative radiology.

Those who are interested in the propagation of knowledge owe a debt of gratitude to Drs. Langlais and Kasle for their industry and efforts in compiling this book. It is greatly to be hoped that they will reap where they have tilled and sowed.

H. M. WORTH, LL.D. Hon. Causa Toronto, F.R.C.P.(C.),
F.R.C.R., F.D.S., R.C.S. Eng.

Preface

This second edition of *Exercises in Oral Radiographic Interpretation* has been a long time coming and we apologize for the delay. We would like to thank all of those individuals who have sent us comments and suggestions for improvement over the past few years. We have seriously attempted to identify the shortcomings of the first edition, and every effort has been made to meet the perceived needs. Although we have expanded the scope of the content of this second edition, we have also eliminated some forty or so cases to make room for the new material. We hope we didn't remove too many of your favorite cases. In this edition we have also re-organized the material in two ways: firstly we have separated dental anomalies and defects from disorders of the jaws, so that each topic is now covered in its own section. Secondly we have grouped related or look-alike disorders within a section to allow for more immediate comparisons and separation of similar but distinctly different conditions. We have also added occlusal, panoramic, and extraoral views in various sections. We have also expanded the localization section to include the use of panoramic films. The last section is an entirely new feature. The National and many State Board Examinations as well as some dental schools have incorporated prints of actual radiographs as a part of their testing process. The multiple-choice format is often used, and this section should serve as an excellent review in the preparation for such examinations.

As you read through this book, don't forget that we have repeated certain conditions or items by design—you should not rule out a certain choice just because it has already been asked. Repetition serves to provide the reader with feedback on what has been learned, and remember, repetition is in itself an enhancement of the learning process! Note also that many clues are given in the question as a part of the history or demographic data about the patient—even in the name! By the way . . . all of the names of the patients given in this book are fictitious.

ROBERT LANGLAIS
MYRON KASLE

Acknowledgments

The authors wish to express their appreciation to the following individuals for their assistance with this manuscript: Denyse Langlais for her constant support and encouragement and for typing the preliminary manuscript; Mr. Richard Scott, Director of Dental Illustrations, Indiana University School of Dentistry, and his staff, Mike Halloran and Alana Fears, for the illustrations; Dr. Rolando De Castro for the masterful artwork in Section 6; the following staff members of the Radiology Department of Indiana University School of Dentistry: Gail Williamson, R.D.H., Carol Ann Steinmetz, and Rosalie Pollack; and the following for allowing us to use certain radiographs: Drs. Carson Mader, Sam Eitner, Tom McDavid, Monique Michaud, Ed. Shields, William Goebel, Malcolm Boone II, Steven Bricker, Robert Hampshire, Jim Cottone, David Blair, Birgit Junfin Glass, Dale Miles, Gus Pappas, and Margot VanDis. The authors would also like to thank Rebecca Cox for her herculean efforts in typing the manuscript for the second edition and Mr. Ray Aldrete of the UTHSCSA Department of Educational Resources for the excellent photographic prints which were added to this edition. Without the assistance of all these individuals this second edition would have been an impossible task.

Preface
to the First Edition

The areas of oral diagnosis and radiology are basic to proper dental patient diagnosis and treatment planning. Visual clinical examination and correct radiographic interpretation correlated with the patient's history and appropriate laboratory values are all necessary to achieve excellence in patient diagnosis and treatment.

We have attempted herein to meet the needs of both students and practitioners with this question-and-answer format. Note that in many cases, certain laboratory values, significant data from the medical, dental, or social history, or the patient's symptoms are given. Use these clues to achieve first the differential diagnosis, and then, with the information given, try to arrive at a substantive working or final diagnosis. When the information contained in the radiographic picture is considered pathognomonic for a certain condition, then no further information other than the radiograph should be required to make the diagnosis. We have included exercises on the identification of normal landmarks as well as possible film artifacts. A knowledge of these areas is essential if accurate diagnosis of disease is to be made and must be acquired if one is to achieve continuing excellence in clinical technique. We have included exercises in the use of the "buccal object rule" because although the principle is simple, its application, if not understood, often generates confusion for the "student" of radiology. We hope that these exercises are the "practice that makes perfect" and will serve as a handy reference on occasions when the buccal object rule is to be used.

In making the differential diagnosis, be certain that the conditions that you select are defendable. In other words, if the lesion is five centimeters in diameter, do not select a lesion that rarely exceeds one centimeter. If the location is in the maxillary cuspid area, do not select a condition that usually occurs in the mandibular molar-ramus area. If the radiograph shows a multilocular radiolucency, do not include entities that are usually unilocular. Select the most commonly occurring lesions with their usual appearance, location, symptoms, and treatment.

The reader should keep in mind that the radiographs are mounted as if viewed from the outside, looking into the oral cavity. The convexity of the film identification dot is facing you.

Well, we hope that you enjoy testing yourself with these selected exercises. You may be pleasantly surprised to find that your knowledge is high; conversely, you may also learn how much you've forgotten! We think that learning should be fun, and we hope you enjoy this learning experience.

R. L.
M. K.

Contents

Section 1
NORMAL ANATOMIC STRUCTURES..................................... 1

Section 2
FILM EXPOSURE AND PROCESSING ERRORS 19

Section 3
IDENTIFICATION OF MATERIALS AND FOREIGN OBJECTS........ 45

Section 4
DEVELOPMENTAL AND ACQUIRED DEFECTS OF THE TEETH.... 57

Section 5
LESIONS AFFECTING THE JAWS 93

Section 6
LOCALIZATION TECHNIQUES... 127

Section 7
REVIEW QUESTIONS FOR NATIONAL AND STATE BOARD
EXAMINATIONS... 135

ANSWERS.. 155

INDEX 193

section 1

Normal Anatomic Structures

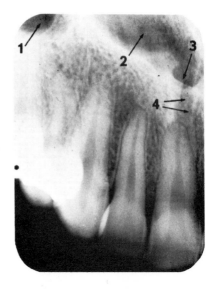

FIGURE 1–1

What entities are the arrows pointing at?

1) maxillary sinus
2) nasal fossa
3) superior foramen of incisive canal
4) incisive canal

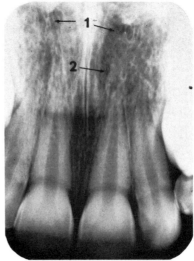

FIGURE 1–2

The arrows are pointing at what entities?

1) sup. foramen of incisive canal

2) incisive canal

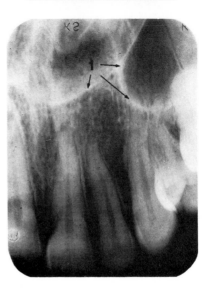

FIGURE 1–3

What is the common name used for this anatomic landmark, and what are the structures that make it up?

floor of nasal fossa & maxillary sinus
are the arms of Y   body is bone

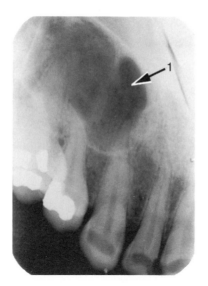

FIGURE 1–4

1. What does the round radiolucent area in this radiograph represent?
2. What could it be misdiagnosed as?

1) sinus recess

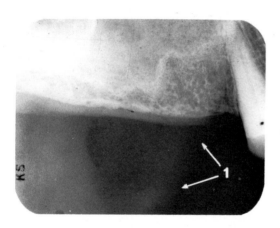

FIGURE 1–5

The border of what entity is indicated by the arrows?

1) nasolabial fold

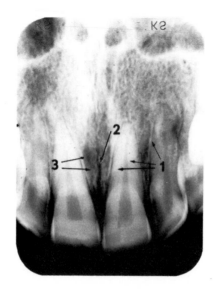

FIGURE 1–6

The arrows are pointing at what commonly recognized structures?

1) the nose
2) median palatal suture
3) incisive foramen

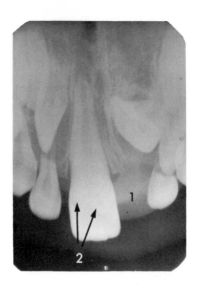

FIGURE 1–7

When the dentist wishes to see this structure, the x-ray exposure should be decreased. What is this structure?

1) Tip of nose
2) peripheral outline of the nose

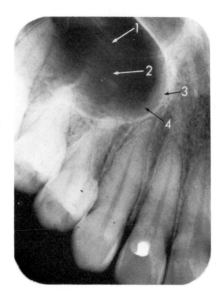

FIGURE 1–8

Entity 1 is commonly found in the wall of entity 2. Entity 3 is often seen outlining entity 2. Entity 4 lines entity 3.

Name the entities indicated in this radiograph.

1) a nutrient canal

2) maxillary sinus

3) cortical plate of the and. wall of max sinus

4) maxillary antral mucosa

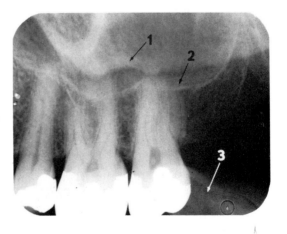

FIGURE 1–9

This view of the maxillary tuberosity area normally contains what entities?

1) zygomatic arch

2) maxillary sinus (floor

3) coronoid process of mandible

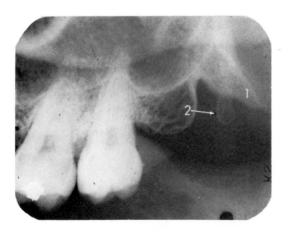

FIGURE 1-10

What do we see in this view?

1) lateral plate of pterygoid processes

2) medial plate of pterygoid processes (hamulus)

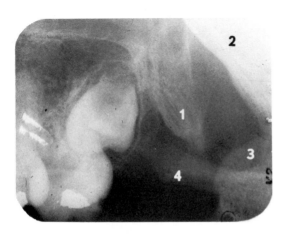

FIGURE 1-11

Viewing the maxillary tuberosity from an extremely posterior position gives one an opportunity to see structures not commonly visible on this intraoral film. See if you can name them without looking at the answer page.

1) pterygoid complex

2) temporal bone

3) mandibular condyle

4) zygomatic arch

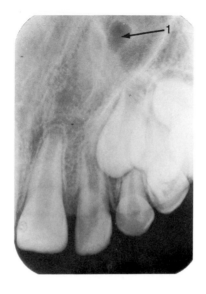

FIGURE 1-12

What entity does this periapical view show?

1) nasolacrimal duct

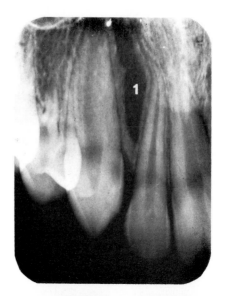

FIGURE 1–13

1. What is the radiolucent area seen between the maxillary lateral incisor and cuspid called?

2. What is it sometimes misdiagnosed as?

1) lateral fossa

2) globulomaxillary cyst

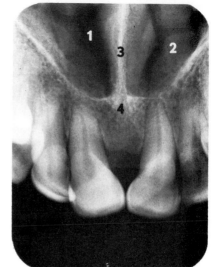

FIGURE 1–14

What radiographic images does this maxillary periapical view demonstrate?

1) nasal fossa

2) inferior turbinate

3) nasal septum

4) anterior nasal spine

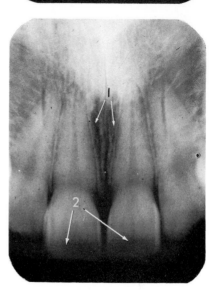

FIGURE 1–15

What does this radiograph demonstrate?

1) incisive foramen

2) upper lip line

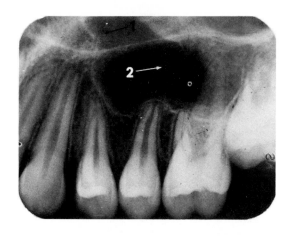

FIGURE 1-16

What do the arrows point at?

1) nasal fossa

2) maxillary sinus

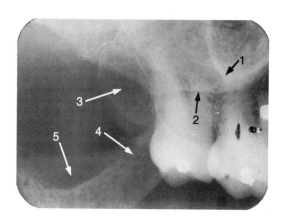

FIGURE 1-17

Identify the structures indicated in this radiograph.

1) zygomatic process of maxilla

2) inf. border of zygomatic arch

3) maxillary tuberosity

4) coronoid process of mandible

5) medial sigmoid depression

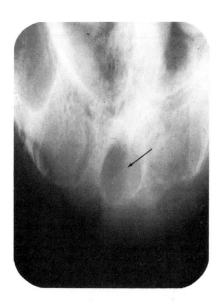

FIGURE 1-18

The arrow is pointing to a maxillary landmark that is occasionally incorrectly identified. What is the name of the landmark, and what is it sometimes incorrectly called?

1) incisive foramen

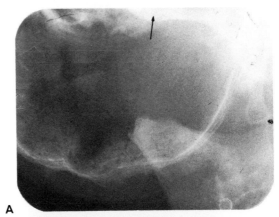

A

FIGURE 1–19

In radiograph *A*, the zygomatic arch is seen at the top of the picture. In radiograph *B*, the zygomatic arch is seen in the middle right of the picture. Explain the differences in these two films.

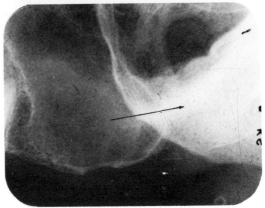

B

FIGURE 1–20

What anatomic landmarks does this view of an edentulous patient demonstrate?

1) zygomatic process of ~~mandible~~ *max*

2) soft tissue shadow of hamular notch

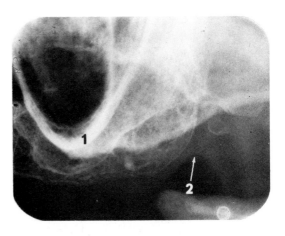

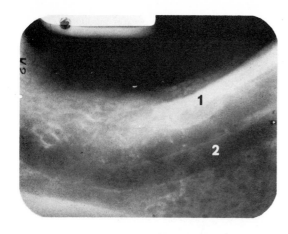

FIGURE 1-21

What are the two commonly seen anatomic landmarks?

1) External oblique ridgue

2) mandibular canal

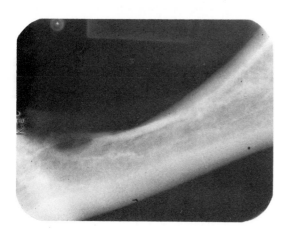

FIGURE 1-22

What is the radiolucency seen on the crest of the ridge?

mental foramen

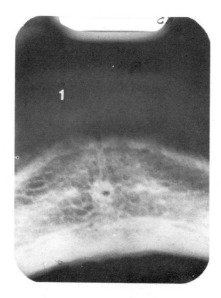

FIGURE 1-23

The first thing to do is to identify the area you're looking at. When you've done that, identify (1) and the round radiopaque area in the center of the bone. What is the small radiolucency in the center of this round radiopaque area?

1) shadow of lower lip

2) round radiopaque area is genial tubercle

radiolucency in center is lingual foramen

FIGURE 1-24

1. What does the radiolucency at the apex of the first bicuspid represent?
2. What does the radiolucent area apical to the first molar represent?

1) mental foramen
2) submandibular fosa

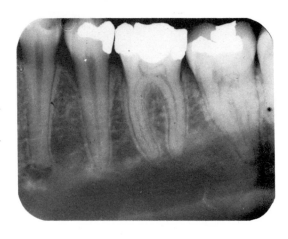

FIGURE 1-25

What are the vertical radiolucent lines viewed on this radiograph?

nutrient canals

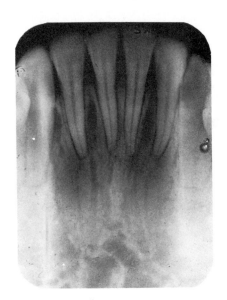

FIGURE 1-26

Identify the structures indicated by the arrows.

1) inferior cortex of mand.

2) submandibular fossa

3) The mand. (inf. alveolar canal)

4) Internal oblique ridge
   (mylohyoid line)

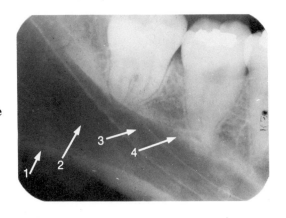

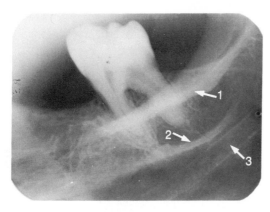

FIGURE 1-27

Name the structures indicated by the arrows.

1) *External oblique ridge*

2) *external oblique ridge*

3) *mandibular inferior alveolar canal*

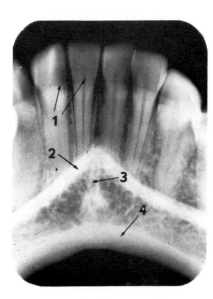

FIGURE 1-28

Beginning at the top, list the areas indicated by the arrows.

1) *lower lip line*

2) *mental ridge*

3) *lingual canal*

4) *cortical plate lower border of the mandible*

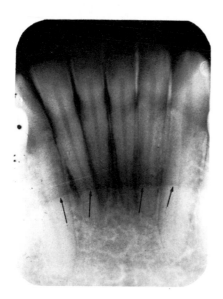

FIGURE 1-29

The arrows are pointing at an anatomic structure that is not usually seen on a periapical radiograph. What is this structure?

anterior border of tongue

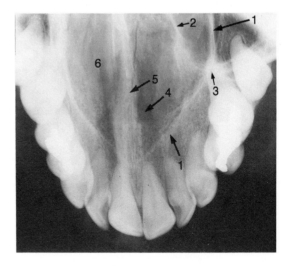

FIGURE 1–30

Name the structures indicated by the arrows and numbers. What radiographic view is this?

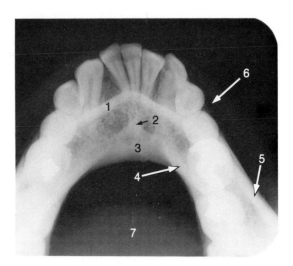

FIGURE 1–31

Name the structures indicated by the arrows and numbers. What is this radiographic view?

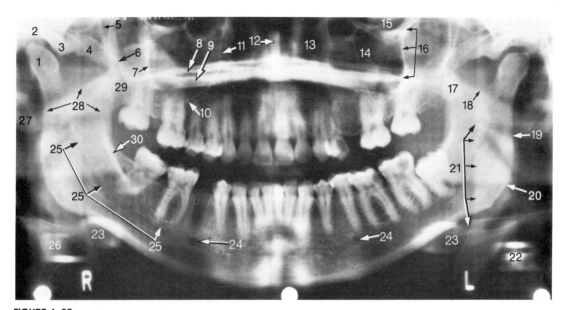

FIGURE 1–32

Name the structures indicated by the numbers and the numbered arrows.

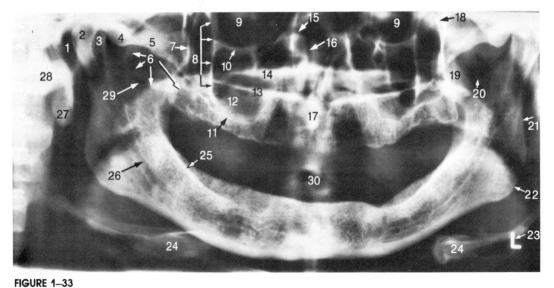

FIGURE 1–33

Name the structures indicated by the numbers and numbered arrows.

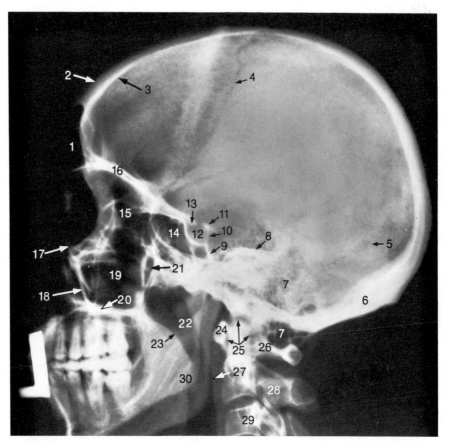

FIGURE 1–34 LATERAL VIEW OF THE SKULL

Name the structures indicated by the numbers and numbered arrows.

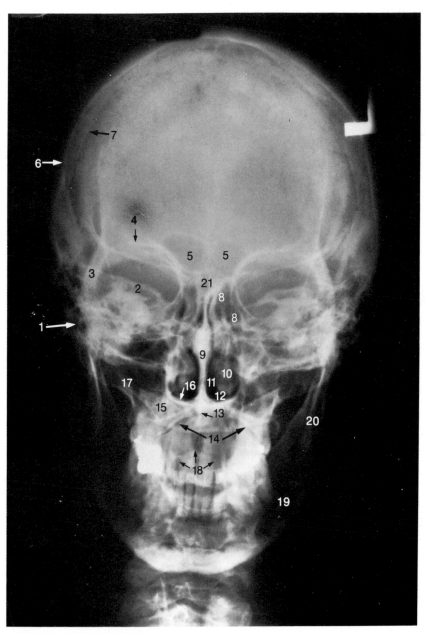

FIGURE 1–35 POSTERO-ANTERIOR VIEW OF THE SKULL

Identify the structures indicated by the numbers and numbered arrows.

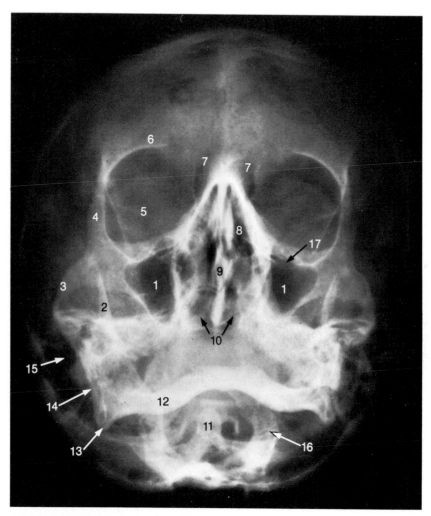

FIGURE 1–36 WATERS' VIEW OF THE SKULL

Name the structures indicated by the numbers and numbered arrows.

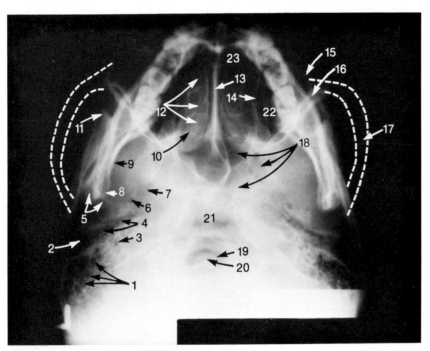

FIGURE 1–37 SUBMENTOVERTEX VIEW OF THE SKULL

Identify the structures indicated by the numbers and numbered arrows. Why does structure No. 17 not show?

Film Exposure and Processing Errors

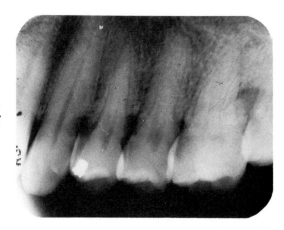

FIGURE 2–1

What is your explanation of the radiolucency seen mainly in the cervical area of the maxillary cuspid and first bicuspid teeth? What causes this?

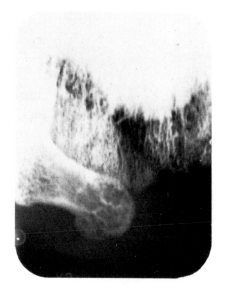

FIGURE 2–2

What term, coined by Dr. David F. Mitchell of Indiana University School of Dentistry, describes the film-handling error seen in this radiograph?

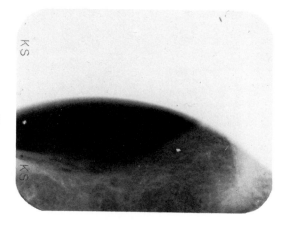

FIGURE 2–3

1. What exposure error was made here?
2. Identify the two small radiopaque spots seen on this film.

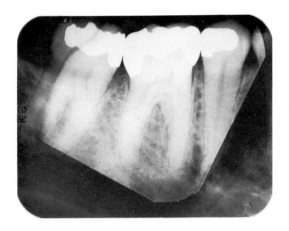

FIGURE 2–4

What film-handling error was made here?

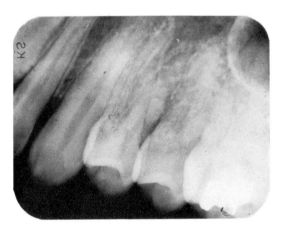

FIGURE 2–5

Why do the roots of the bicuspid teeth appear "fuzzed out"?

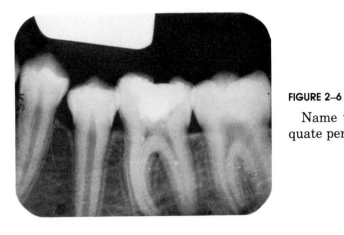

FIGURE 2–6

Name two possible causes for the inadequate periapical coverage.

FIGURE 2-7

How can a "blank" image such as this be produced?

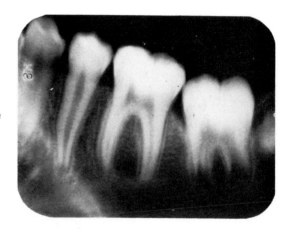

FIGURE 2-8

What exposure error or errors may have been made here?

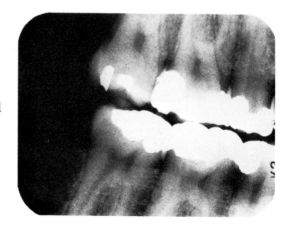

FIGURE 2-9

1. How would you describe the overall appearance of this radiograph?
2. How does this occur?

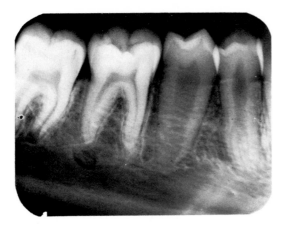

FIGURE 2–10

What processing solution can produce the artifact seen at the apex of the mandibular first molar?

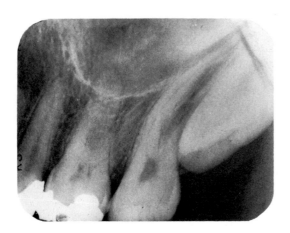

FIGURE 2–11

What film-handling error was made here?

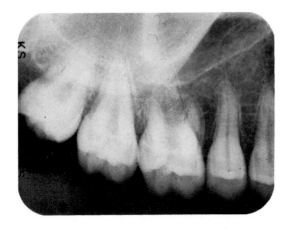

FIGURE 2–12

1. What exposure error was made?
2. What was the cause?

FIGURE 2–13

What film-handling error was made here?

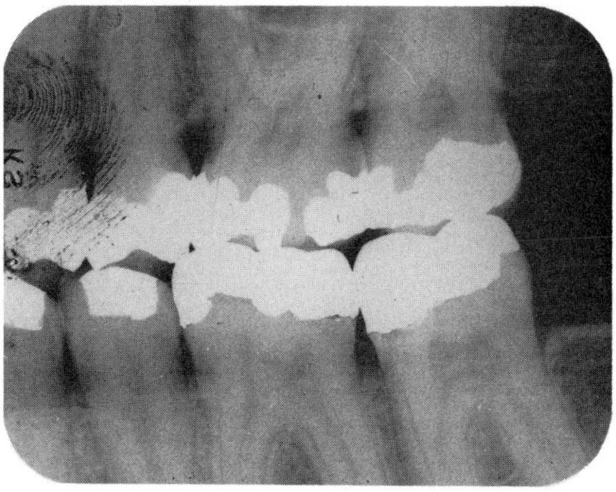

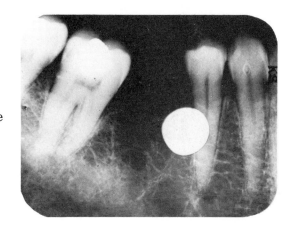

FIGURE 2–14

What processing solution may produce this artifact?

FIGURE 2–15

Now, tell us what exposure error was made here.

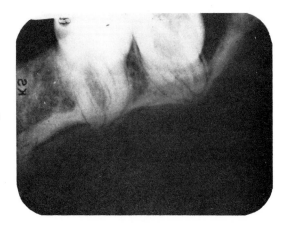

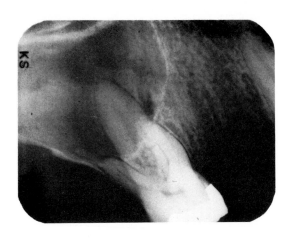

FIGURE 2–16

Why does the palatal root appear to be so much longer than the mesial buccal and distal buccal roots of this maxillary molar?

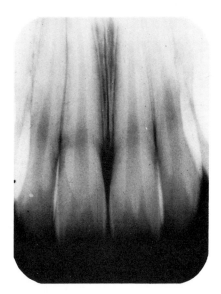

FIGURE 2–17

What error was made? Explain your answer.

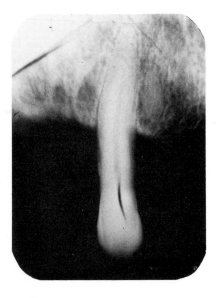

FIGURE 2–18

Can you name two film errors evident in this radiograph? Yes, you can. Try.

FIGURE 2–19

What exposure error has been made here? How?

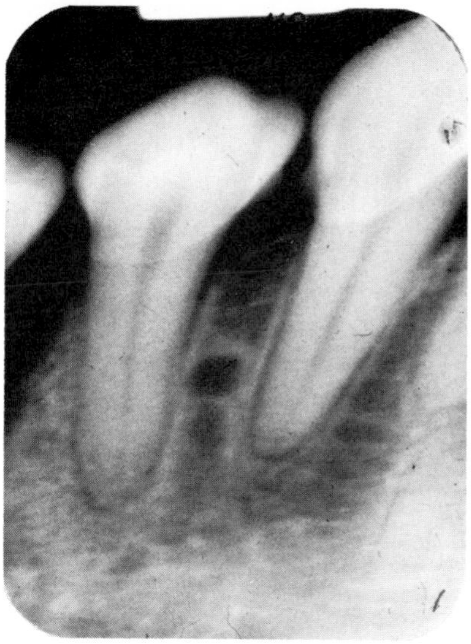

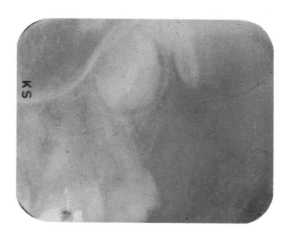

FIGURE 2–20

List some reasons why this film is too light.

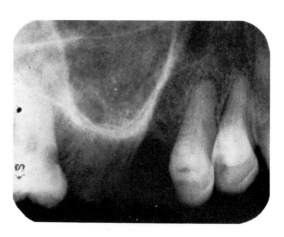

FIGURE 2–21

1. What anatomic structure is superimposed over the entire crown and root of the maxillary molar?

2. How did this superimposition occur?

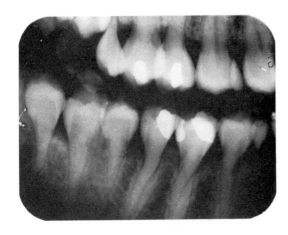

FIGURE 2–22

What exposure error was made?

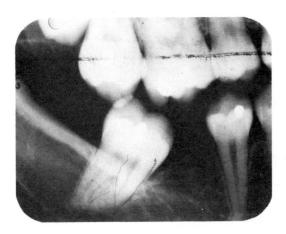

FIGURE 2–23

What do you suppose produced the horizontal black line across the crowns of the maxillary teeth in this radiograph developed by automatic film-processing methods?

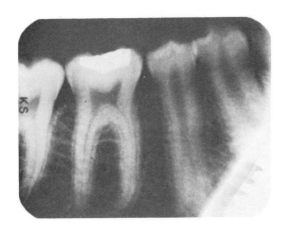

FIGURE 2–24

Give a commentary on the white line seen in the lower right-hand corner of this film.

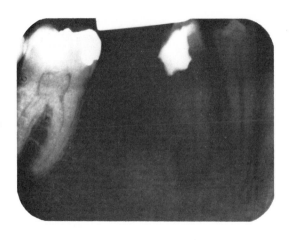

FIGURE 2–25

List possible reasons why this film is too dark.

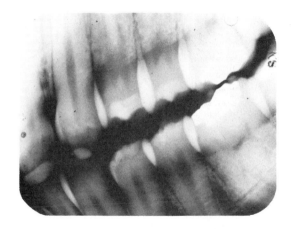

FIGURE 2–26

What technical error was made? How?

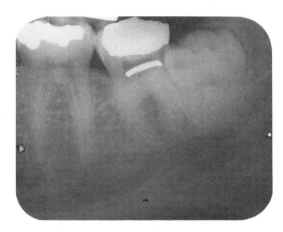

FIGURE 2–27

What film-handling error produced this radiopaque artifact over the second molar?

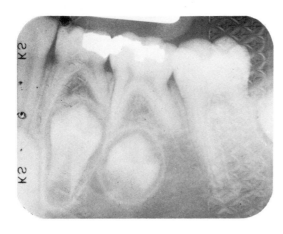

FIGURE 2–28

What film-handling error was made?

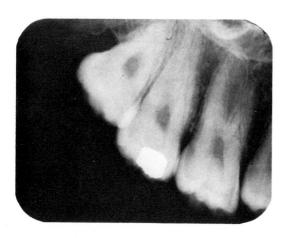

FIGURE 2–29

Why were the apices of the second and third maxillary molars missed?

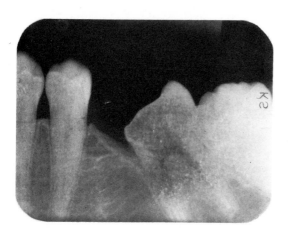

FIGURE 2–30

What processing error was made? (Clinically the film looked a little greenish.)

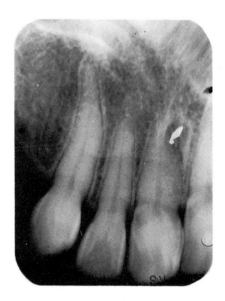

FIGURE 2–31

List possible reasons why this film was fogged.

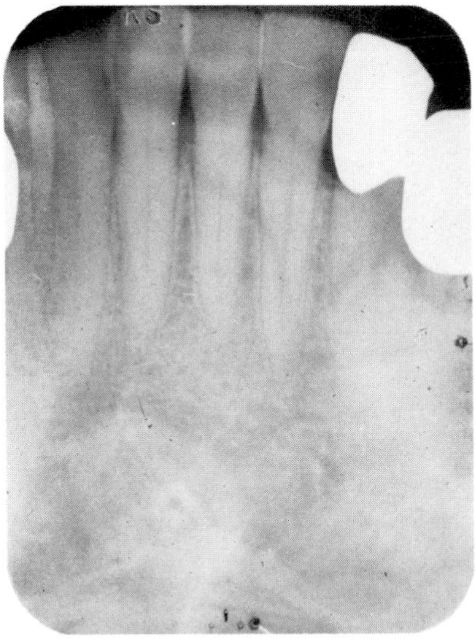

FIGURE 2–32

Give your differential diagnosis of the condition represented by the radiopaque portion of the periapical radiolucency seen in this radiograph. Include possible artifacts.

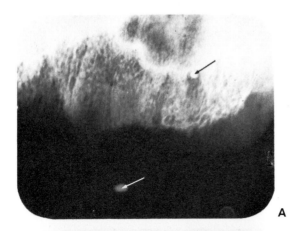

A

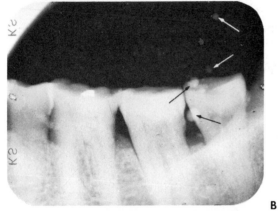

B

FIGURE 2–33

The radiopaque circular areas in these three radiographs are all of different origins. What is your list of possible causes of these opacities (arrows)?

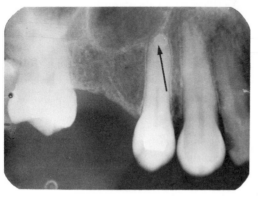

C

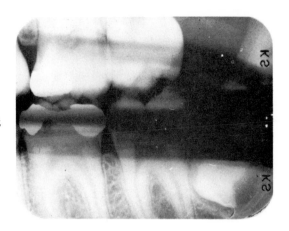

FIGURE 2–34

What film-processing artifact is present here?

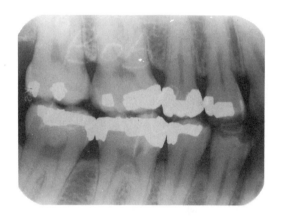

FIGURE 2–35

What happened to this film?

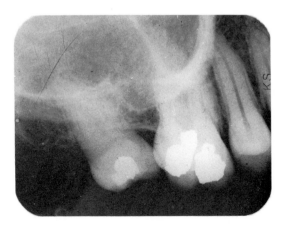

FIGURE 2–36

1. What anatomic structure superimposed on the maxillary antrum is causing the sinus to appear cloudy, as if fluid-filled?

2. What exposure error produced this effect?

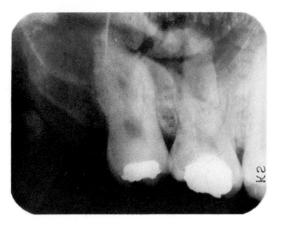

FIGURE 2–37

This radiograph was processed in solutions at 90°F; the film was then rinsed under the cold-water tap. Give the term for what happens to the emulsion when this film-processing error is made.

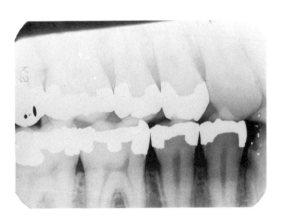

FIGURE 2–38

This film was correctly exposed. The upper dark area looked greenish clinically. Name or describe two manual processing errors that occurred.

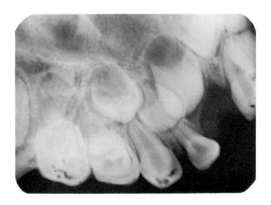

FIGURE 2–39

What artifact, which mimics enamel hypoplasia, is present in this radiograph of deciduous teeth?

FIGURE 2–40

The artifact seen on this radiograph resembles a fistulous tract. What is this artifact?

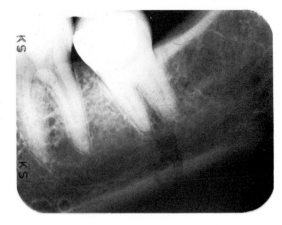

FIGURE 2–41

What film-handling or processing errors are evident here?

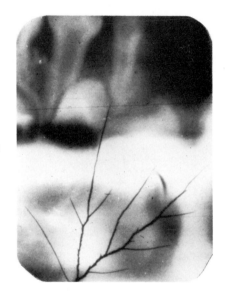

FIGURE 2–42

What exposure error occurred here? Hint: a collimating device was used.

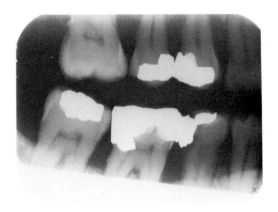

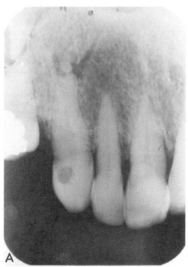

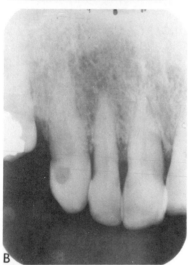

FIGURE 2–43

Films A and B came from the same double packet. Film A's image, however, differs from that of Film B. What error or artifact—if any—affecting Film A would account for this?

1. Fixer artifact
2. Developer artifact
3. Scratched emulsion
4. There is neither an error nor an artifact present here (and there is essentialy no real difference between the films).

FIGURE 2–44

Look at these two films carefully. Both came from the same double packet, but they are not necessarily identical. What artifact or error—if any—can be seen that would account for this?

1. There are no signs of an artifact or error, and there is no real difference between the films.

2. Fluoride stain

3. Developer artifact

4. Fixer artifact

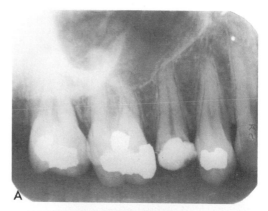

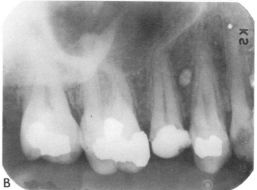

FIGURE 2–45

What technical error—if any—occurred here?

1. Foreshortening

2. There was no error; this case represents hereditary rootless teeth.

3. Denture with plastic teeth was left in.

4. Denture with porcelain teeth was left in.

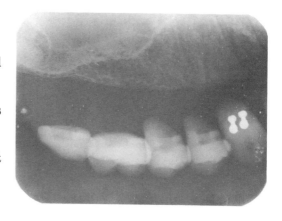

FIGURES 2–46 THROUGH 2–51

In each of the following six panoramic films, a patient positioning error was made. For each film:

1. Name the patient positioning error.
2. Identify the specific findings on each film that identify the error.

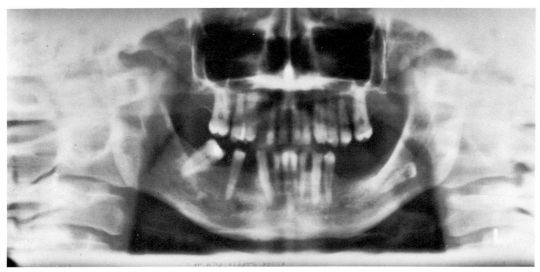

FIGURE 2–46

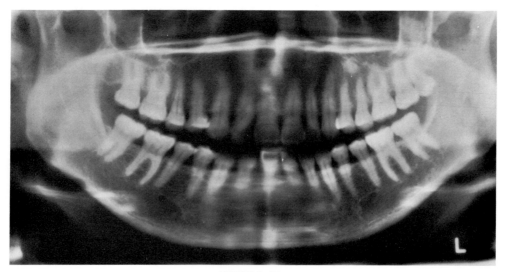

FIGURE 2–47

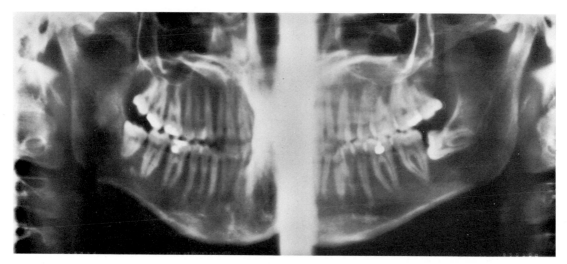

FIGURE 2–48

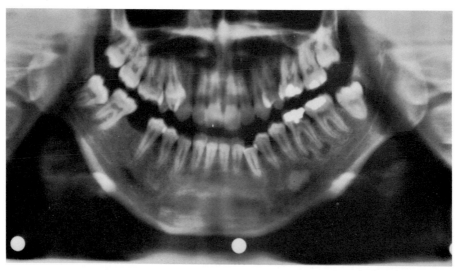

FIGURE 2–49

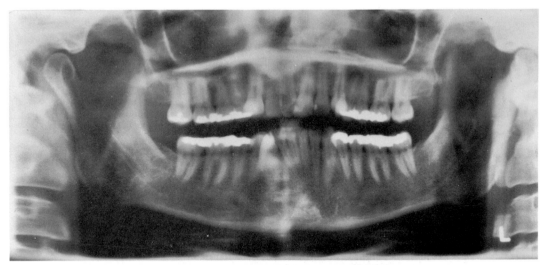

FIGURE 2–50

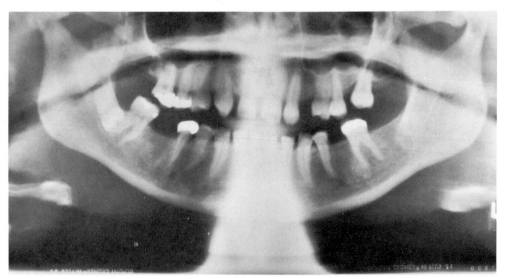

FIGURE 2–51

In each of the following six panoramic films, an operator-related procedural error was made. For each film:

1. Name the procedural error.
2. Describe the altered image characteristics due to the error.

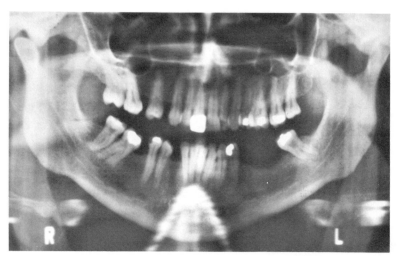

FIGURE 2–52

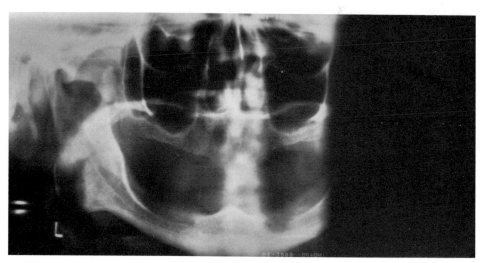

FIGURE 2–53

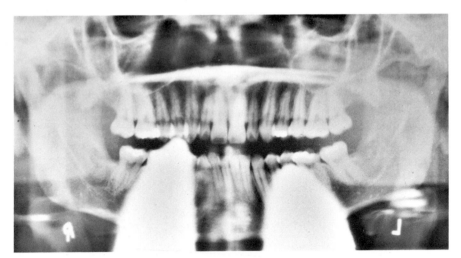

FIGURE 2–54

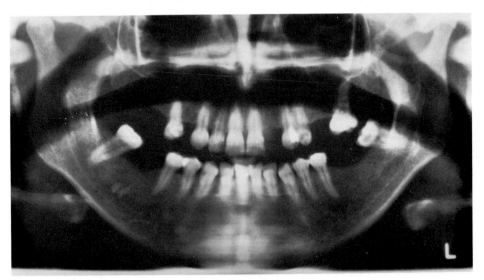

FIGURE 2–55

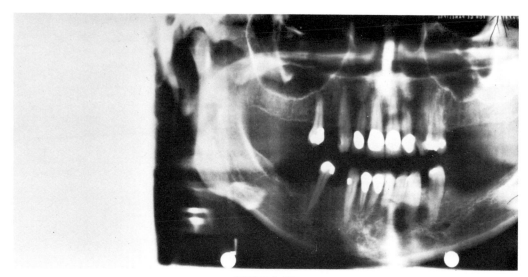

FIGURE 2–56

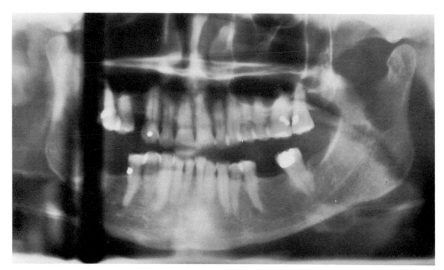

FIGURE 2–57

Identification of Materials and Foreign Objects

FIGURE 3–1

1. What materials could have been used to restore the mesial of the central incisors?

2. What materials could have been used to restore the distal of the central incisors?

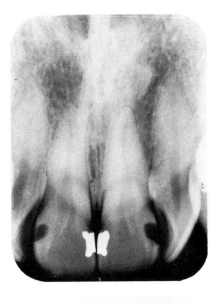

FIGURE 3–2

1. With what metals might this patient's prosthesis be made?

2. With what material are the crowns of the anterior teeth restored?

3. What are the radiopaque lines seen in the cervical area of the anterior teeth?

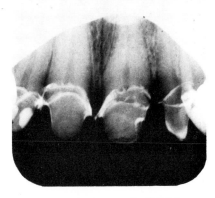

FIGURE 3–3

What type of crown has been placed on the right central incisor?

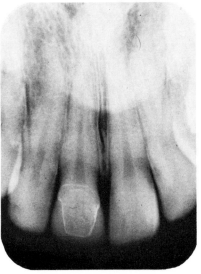

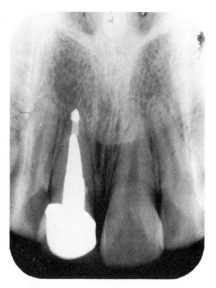

FIGURE 3–4

What restorative materials have been used to treat the right central incisor?

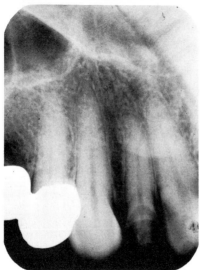

FIGURE 3–5

What material has been used to restore the crown of the lateral incisor?

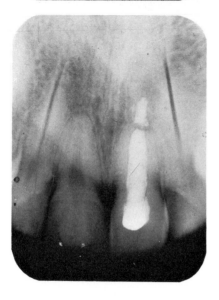

FIGURE 3–6

1. What material has been used to restore the crown of the right central incisor?

2. What might the two radiopaque dots represent?

3. What other materials are seen in this radiograph?

4. What is the cause of the radiolucent lines at the upper corners of this film?

FIGURE 3–7

This case involves a 23 year old patient who presented for a routine examination. The full-mouth radiographic survey revealed a radiopaque object on the cervical third of the root of the left central incisor. There was no restoration on this tooth, and it was vital. There was no history of pain. With careful questioning, the patient revealed that she had been involved in an automobile accident several months earlier.

1. What is your most likely diagnosis of this radiopacity?

2. What are some other circumstances or objects that might produce a similar radiographic picture?

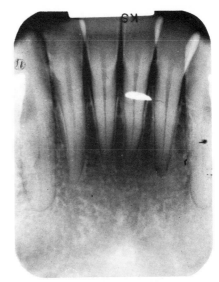

FIGURE 3–8

1. What is the approximate age of this patient? How do you know?

2. Is the right central incisor in lingual or labial version? Give the reason for your answer.

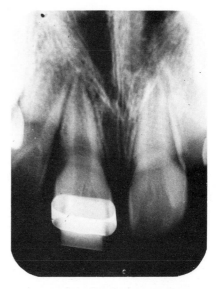

FIGURE 3–9

1. What is the name of the appliance seen in this radiograph?

2. Does this appear to be a young or elderly patient? Give the reason for your answer.

3. What was the probable reason for initiating this type of therapy?

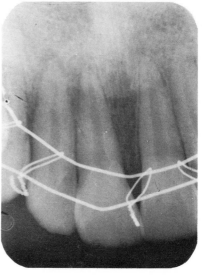

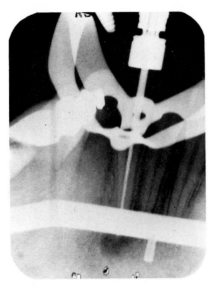

FIGURE 3–10

Name five metallic objects that can be identified in this radiograph.

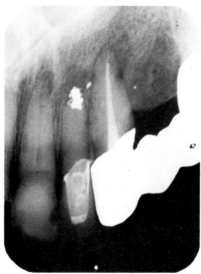

FIGURE 3–11

1. What two forms of endodontic therapy may be seen in this radiograph?

2. Give two reasons why the lateral incisor was not treated in a manner similar to that used to treat the cuspid.

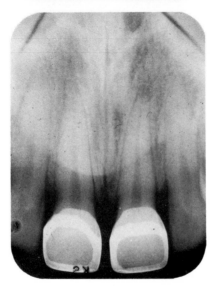

FIGURE 3–12

With what material are the central incisors restored?

Viewing from left to right, tell what materials the arrows are pointing to in each of the following radiographs.

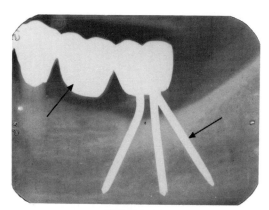

FIGURE 3–13

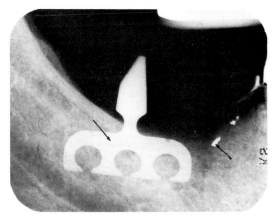

FIGURE 3–14

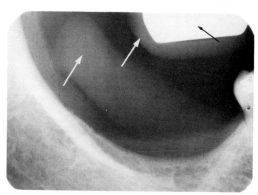

FIGURE 3–15

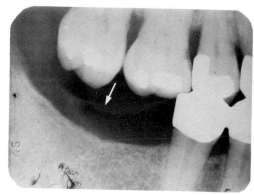

FIGURE 3–16

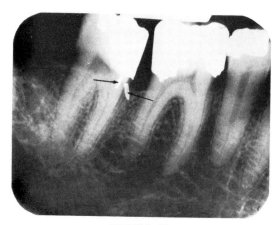

FIGURE 3–17

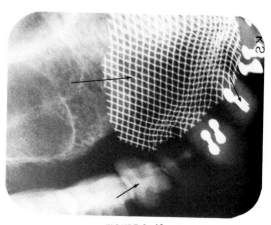

FIGURE 3–18

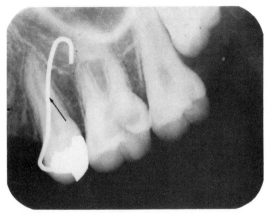

FIGURE 3–19

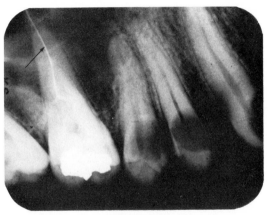

FIGURE 3–20

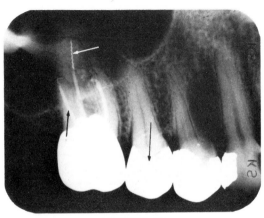

FIGURE 3–21

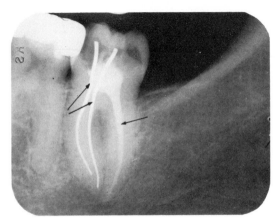

FIGURE 3–22

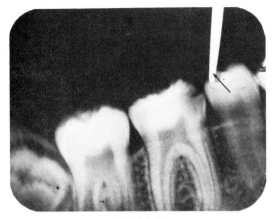

FIGURE 3–23

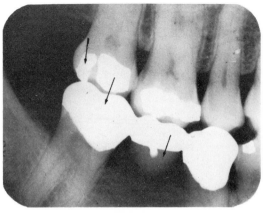

FIGURE 3–24

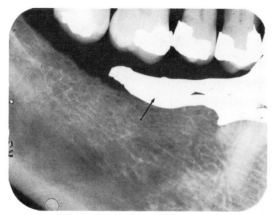

FIGURE 3–25

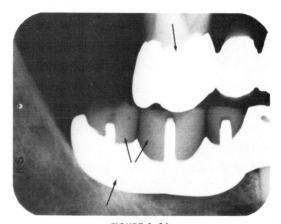

FIGURE 3–26

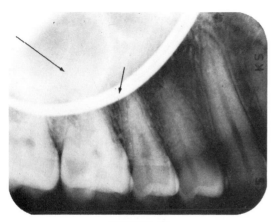

FIGURE 3–27

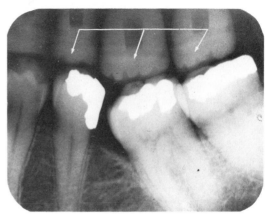

FIGURE 3–28

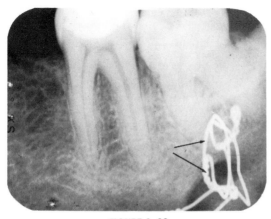

FIGURE 3–29

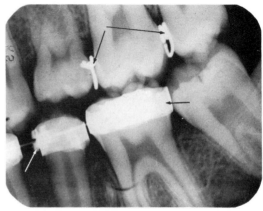

FIGURE 3–30

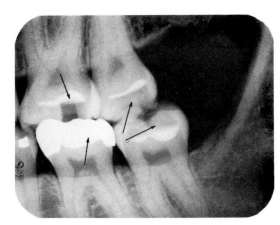

FIGURE 3–31

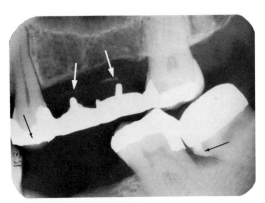

FIGURE 3–32

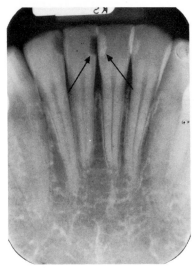

FIGURE 3–33

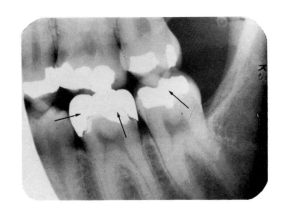

FIGURE 3–34

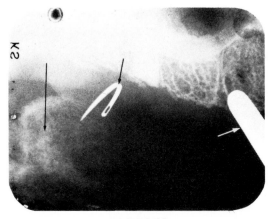

FIGURE 3–35

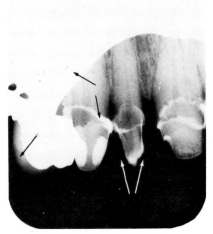

FIGURE 3–36

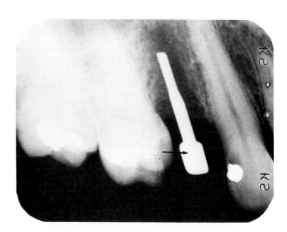

FIGURE 3–37

FIGURE 3–38

What materials were used to restore the mandibular second deciduous molar seen in this radiograph?

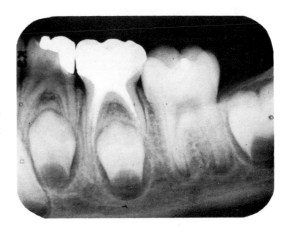

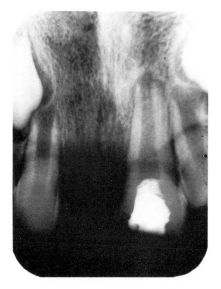

FIGURE 3–39

What material was used in this fractured central incisor?

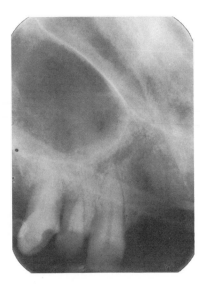

FIGURE 3–40

·An image crossing the apex of these teeth is slightly visible. This patient had difficulty breathing. What might the image represent?

Developmental and Acquired Defects of the Teeth

FIGURE 4–1

1. Name the developmental anomaly in the lateral incisor.
2. What other condition of significance in endodontic treatment planning is present in this tooth?

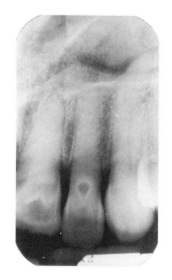

FIGURE 4–2

1. Describe the radiographic appearance of the mandibular first permanent molar seen in this radiograph.
2. What pathologic entities can be seen?

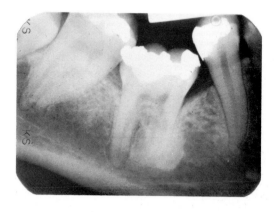

FIGURE 4–3

Johnny Ecto has sparse blond hair and a ruddy-red complexion and is uncomfortable in warm weather. The bridge of his nose is depressed and he has full pouting lips.

1. What hereditary condition does Johnny have?

2. The dental findings in this condition also may be noted in two other disorders; name them.

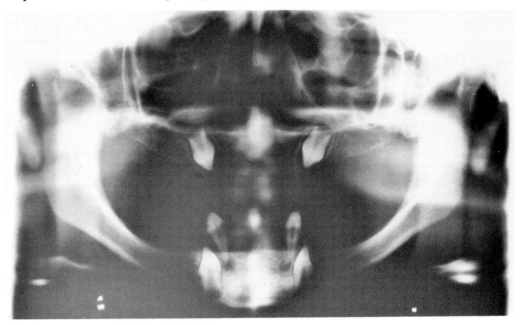

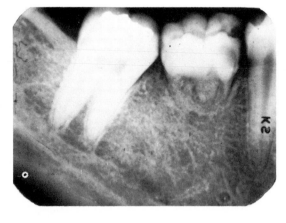

FIGURE 4–4

Mary Sweet, now 24 years old, was involved as a patient in a dental research project when she was 18. Her nontreatable carious mandibular first permanent molar was extracted as part of the overall dental treatment.

1. Based on the radiograph, what do you suppose that treatment procedure was?

2. Describe the radiographic appearance of the tooth occupying the place of the mandibular first molar.

FIGURE 4–5

Clyde Boss is 22 years old and is the life of the party when he demonstrates his ability to hold a glass between his two shoulders. The skull films showed open fontanelles and wormian bones, the result of many open sutures. There was frontal boss-ing and most of the permanent teeth failed to erupt. There were also some supernumerary permanent teeth.

1. Name Clyde's condition.
2. What is different about the roots of the permanent teeth in individuals affected by this condition?

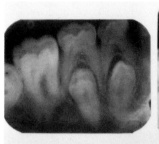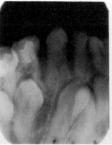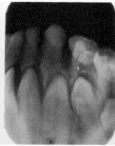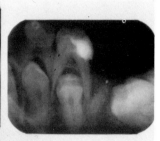

FIGURE 4–6

1. Identify the abnormality in this radiograph.
2. Name one syndrome with which this finding may be associated.
3. What is the importance of recognizing this syndrome in children?

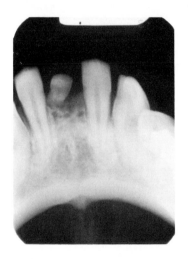

FIGURE 4–7

What three conditions associated with the mandibular second molar would you, as the consulting radiologist, note in this radiograph?

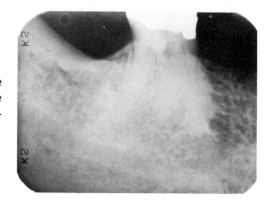

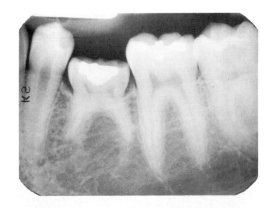

FIGURE 4–8

1. What is the main problem depicted in this radiograph?

2. What notation would you make on the patient's chart regarding the second molar?

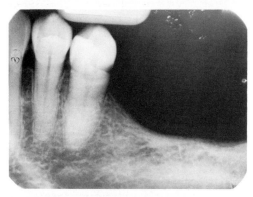

FIGURE 4–9

The features in this radiograph are pathognomonic of what factitial injury to the mandibular second bicuspid?

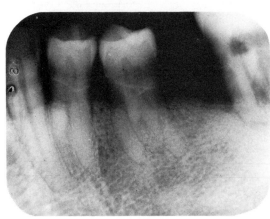

FIGURE 4–10

1. In viewing this radiograph, detail the abnormalities you can discern regarding the following:
    a. the occlusal surfaces,
    b. pulp chambers,
    c. cervical area, and
    d. roots.

2. Name two other periodontally notable pathologic processes seen in this radiograph.

3. What film-handling error was made in the taking of this radiograph?

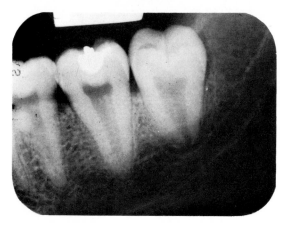

FIGURE 4–11

How would you describe the root shape of the molars in this radiograph?

FIGURE 4-12

1. What term is used to describe the variation in form of the first molar in this radiograph?

2. With what syndromes may this tooth form be associated?

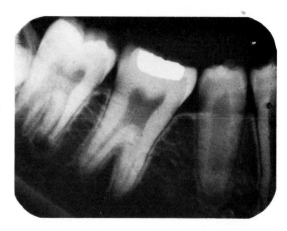

FIGURE 4-13

1. What is the most obvious abnormality seen in this radiograph?

2. Name two conditions with which this abnormality may be associated.

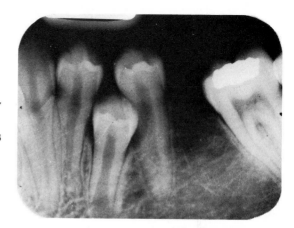

FIGURE 4-14

Belinda Brokenbone is a 24 year old who is confined to a wheelchair; she has had a long history of fractures of the long bones. She has blue eyes—the sclerae of which are also blue—and is very small in stature. Clinically, her teeth appear to have normal shape and size. She has a low caries history. When she smiles, as she often does, her anterior teeth appear to have an opalescent sheen.

1. What is Belinda's systemic condition?

2. What developmental dental defect is involved?

3. What features of this condition are seen radiographically?

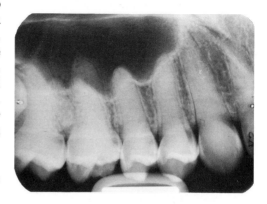

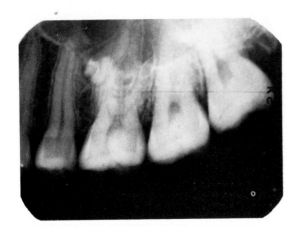

FIGURE 4–15

What unusual entity do you see in this radiograph?

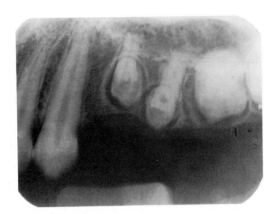

FIGURE 4–16

This case involves a 13 year old female who had Hodgkin's disease at age five. The only manifestations of the disease were low-grade fever and cervical lymphadenopathy that persisted even after three weeks of antibiotic treatment. She received the usual mode of therapy and is presently free of disease.

1. What is the common mode of therapy?
2. What effects did this have on her teeth?

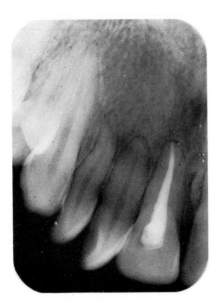

FIGURE 4–17

What developmental anomaly can be clearly seen in this radiograph?

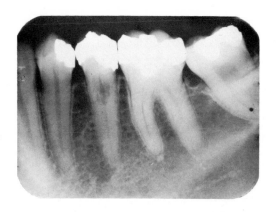

FIGURE 4–18

1. Compare the radiographic appearance of the pulps of the mandibular second bicuspid and the first molar.

2. How would you treat these pulps? Give your reasons for this treatment.

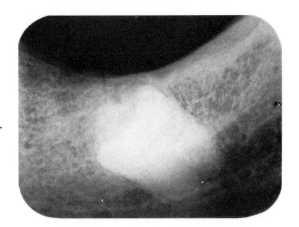

FIGURE 4–19

1. Where is this radiopacity located?

2. What does it represent?

3. What alterations have occurred in association with this radiopacity?

4. How would you treat this?

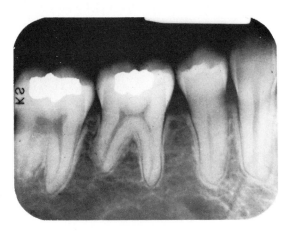

FIGURE 4–20

1. Identify the following radiolucencies:
   a. the crest of the ridge between the second bicuspid and the first molar and
   b. the one near the apex of the second bicuspid.

2. Give the term for the dentistry that was done here and what it brought about. (Note adverse consequences especially.)

3. What other pathological dental finding is evident?

FIGURE 4-21

1. Name the condition that affects these teeth.

2. What are the condition's characteristic features? (Not necessarily all of them are in this radiograph.)

3. How do these teeth look clinically?

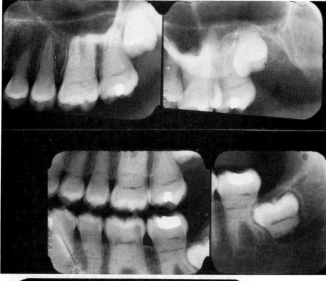

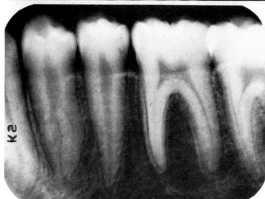

FIGURE 4-22

1. What developmental anomaly do you see here?

2. What structure do the two thin radiolucent lines at the apex of the mesial root of the mandibular first molar represent?

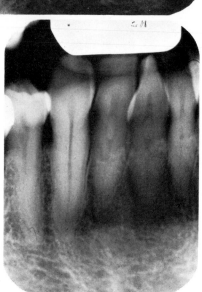

FIGURE 4-23

In reviewing this radiograph, what points of interest should you note?

FIGURE 4-24

Describe and locate the entity represented by the central radiopacity in this radiograph.

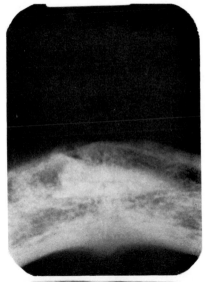

FIGURE 4-25

1. What developmental anomaly is seen here?

2. Would you suspect that this radiopacity is located more palatally or labially?

3. How else could you locate this structure?

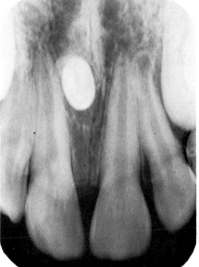

FIGURE 4-26

What term is used to describe this particular set of circumstances?

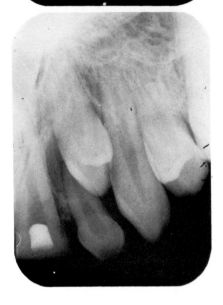

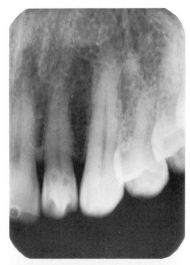

FIGURE 4–27

1. What term is used to describe the clinical appearance of the coronal portion of the lateral incisor?

2. What other anomaly can be seen?

3. What treatment would you recommend?

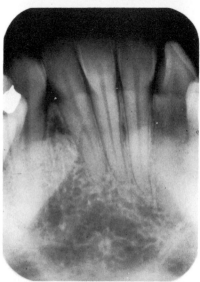

FIGURE 4–28

1. Toward what endodontically significant structure does the radiopacity on the left of the radiograph appear to be pointing?

2. What are these bilateral radiopaque structures?

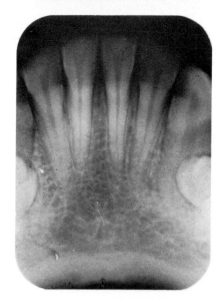

FIGURE 4–29

What would you interpret the bilateral radiopaque structures seen in the lower corners of this radiograph to represent?

After checking your answers, take a break.

Welcome back. Ready to start again? Here we go.

FIGURE 4–30

What structures account for the notched appearance of the mandibular incisor teeth?

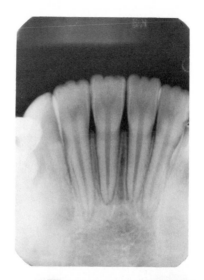

FIGURE 4–31

1. What developmental anomaly can be seen in this radiograph?

2. What are the radiographic signs of this anomaly?

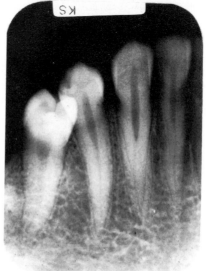

FIGURE 4–32

1. In viewing this radiograph, what notations would you make concerning the maxillary cuspid?

2. What type of restoration was used on this tooth?

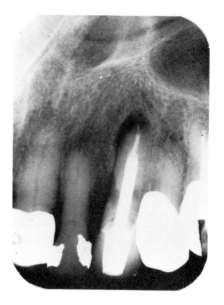

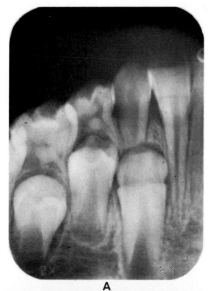

A

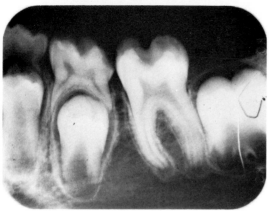

B

FIGURE 4–33

These two radiographs are from the same patient.
1. How old is the patient?
2. What developmental defect is present?
3. What teeth are affected?

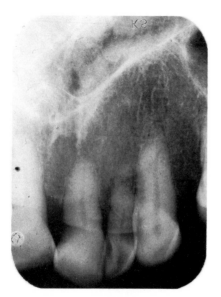

FIGURE 4–34

1. What does the radiopaque line in the cervical area of the central, lateral, and cuspid teeth represent?

2. What technical error was made on this radiograph?

FIGURE 4–35

Julie Eatmore is a healthy 21 year old with a slight weight problem. When you examined her teeth clinically the lingual of the anterior maxillary teeth was shiny and smooth and seemed to have very thin enamel. Sensitivity of the teeth to temperature changes is in fact what brought Julie in for her visit. Although her medical history was non-contributory, she did finally admit that she was receiving psychologic treatment for an "eating disorder."

1. What eating disorder do you suppose she has?

2. What relationship does this disorder have to the teeth?

3. What's wrong with the teeth?

4. What is the term used to describe the appearance of the maxillary anterior teeth?

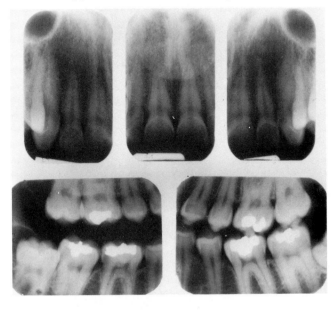

FIGURE 4–36

What term is used to describe the spaces between these teeth?

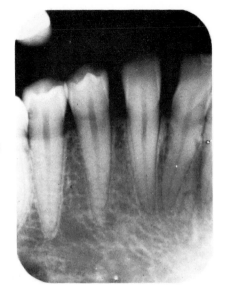

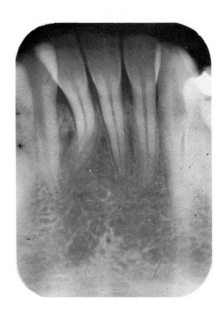

FIGURE 4–37

What term is used to describe the malformation seen in this radiograph?

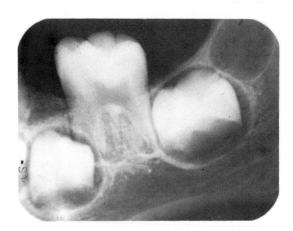

FIGURE 4–38

This patient is seven years old. What is your impression of the radiolucency just distal to the last molar?

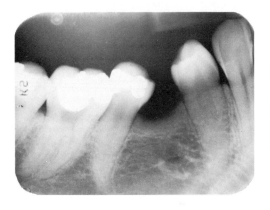

FIGURE 4–39

The only tooth that this patient has ever lost is the right mandibular permanent first molar. What term is used to describe the phenomenon that has occurred here?

FIGURE 4–40

In this case, the patient, now 11 years old, had a history of high fever when he was very young.

1. Estimate within one year the age at which the fever probably occurred.

2. What was the result of this fever?

3. What other teeth, not shown here, could have been affected?

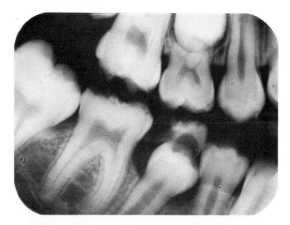

FIGURE 4–41

The patient is a 10 year old boy who just had a recall examination. Although he has no caries in his permanent dentition, he has a history of having an abscessed first deciduous molar, which has just exfoliated.

After viewing this radiograph, what would you report?

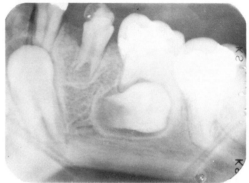

FIGURE 4–42

The features depicted in this radiograph are pathognomonic of what condition?

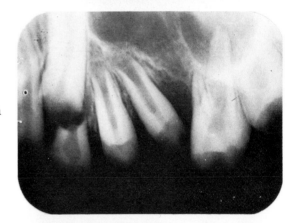

FIGURE 4–43

Detail your impression of:

1. the pontic material,

2. the radiopacity associated with the pontic, and

3. the radiolucency at the apex of the second bicuspid.

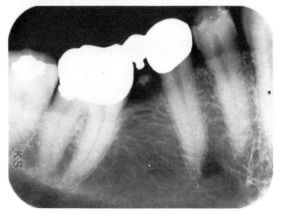

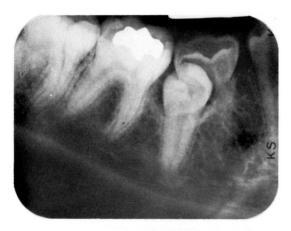

FIGURE 4–44

Will the mandibular second bicuspid erupt?

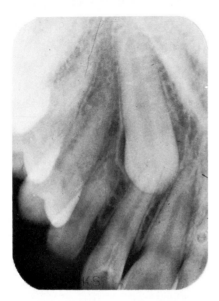

FIGURE 4–45

After viewing this radiograph, what do you report? Be thorough.

FIGURE 4–46

What condition is illustrated in both of these radiographs?

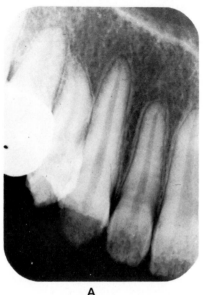

A

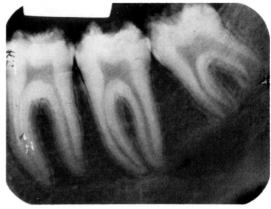

B

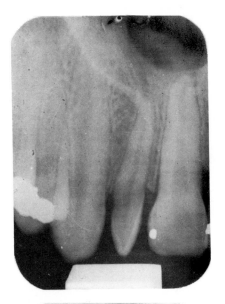

FIGURE 4–47

How would you describe the shape of the maxillary lateral incisor?

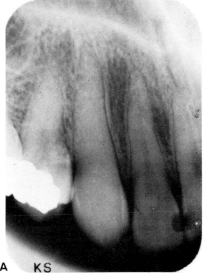

FIGURE 4–48

1. What pulpal condition do these two radiographs demonstrate?

2. What is the significance of this in case A?

3. What is the significance of this in case B?

A   KS

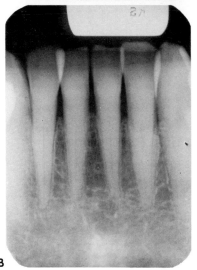

B

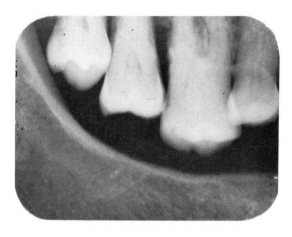

FIGURE 4–49

1. What term is used to describe the relationship of these maxillary molars to the mandibular ridge?

2. Name the two contributing causes.

FIGURE 4–50 through 4–55

The next group of questions relates to caries or to the sequelae of caries.

In each figure there are lettered arrows indicating a surface to be interpreted. For each arrow, select one of the following numbers that you feel most accurately describes the caries.

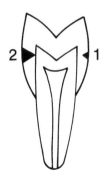

0: *no caries*

1: *incipient caries*; halfway through the enamel or less

2: *early caries*; limited to enamel only

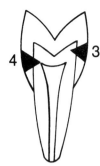

3: *frank caries*; involving the dentinoenamel junction, but less than halfway between the dentin and the pulp

4: *deep caries*; more than halfway through the dentin and/or encroaching upon the pulp

Interpret only the surfaces indicated by the lettered arrows. *Do not interpret the caries as deeper than indicated on the radiograph even if you suspect that clinically the caries may be of greater depth.*

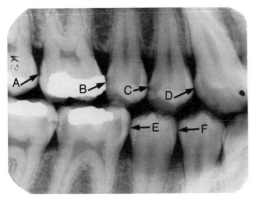

FIGURE 4–50

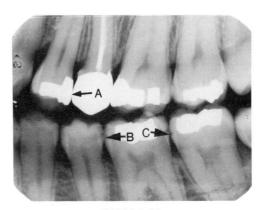

FIGURE 4–51

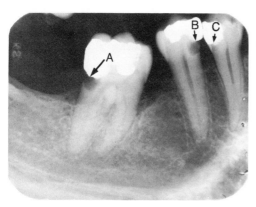

FIGURE 4–52

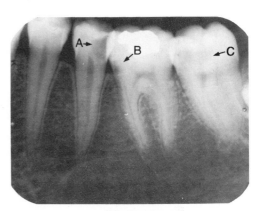

FIGURE 4–53

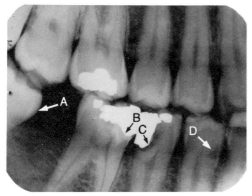

FIGURE 4–54

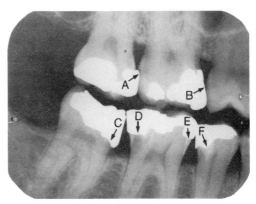

FIGURE 4–55

77

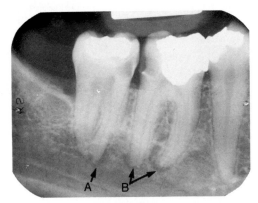

FIGURE 4–56

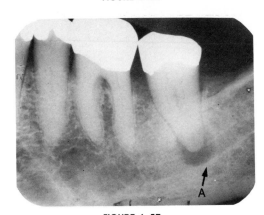

FIGURE 4–57

In each of the following cases a periapical lesion of pulpul origin is indicated by a lettered arrow. For each lettered arrow do the following:

1. Give the radiographic diagnosis or differential diagnosis.

2. State the probable cause of the lesion.

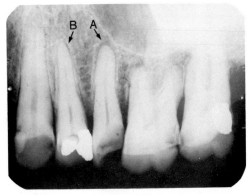

FIGURE 4–58

FIGURE 4–59

Mrs. X is a 35 year old patient who was treated with cobalt 60 for an oral malignancy.

1. What pathologic process is affecting these teeth?

2. Which tooth shows the most typical lesion?

3. Why do these lesions occur?

4. How can this sequela be prevented?

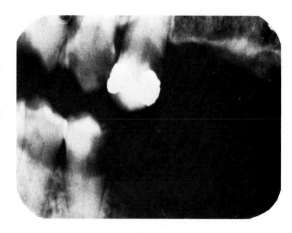

FIGURE 4–60

1. Give a differential diagnosis of the periapical radiolucency seen in this radiograph of a 34 year old black female.

2. What objective test would be of great help in determining the proper treatment of this lesion?

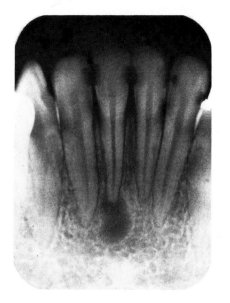

FIGURE 4–61

Compare the radiolucencies seen at the apices of the mandibular first and second molars in this radiograph.

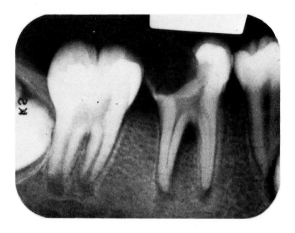

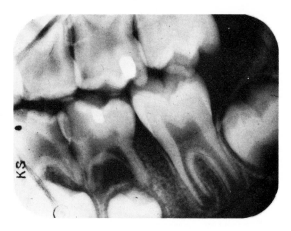

FIGURE 4–62

1. What is the probable cause of the bifurcation involvement of the mandibular second deciduous molar?

2. Can this condition affect the developing permanent tooth?

3. If so, what is this condition?

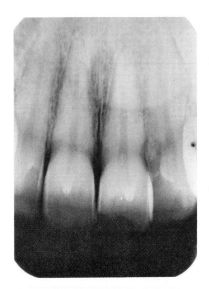

FIGURE 4–63

1. What anatomic structure produces the semicircular radiopacity at the apical third of the root of the left central incisor?

2. What anatomic structure produces the radiopaque line along the incisal third of these anterior teeth?

3. Why may one or more of these teeth be nonvital?

    4. a. What developmental anomaly can be seen in association with the crowns of the central incisor?

       b. What analogous condition may be seen on the occlusal of the mandibular bicuspid teeth of Asians?

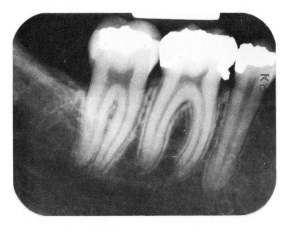

FIGURE 4–64

1. What radiopaque entity is present that may lead to alveolar bone loss?

2. Of the three teeth seen in this radiograph, which one do you suppose would be the most difficult to extract?

FIGURE 4–65

In the event of caries, would the bicuspid teeth seen in this radiograph be more susceptible to an early pulpitis than normally? Give the reason for your answer.

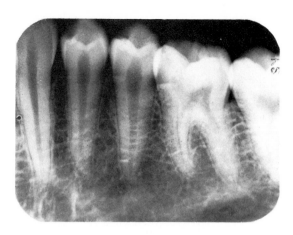

FIGURE 4–66

Name two developmental anomalies that can be seen to be developing in this radiograph.

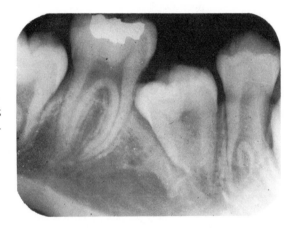

FIGURE 4–67

Relative to the size of the teeth seen in this radiograph, what term is used to describe this developmental condition?

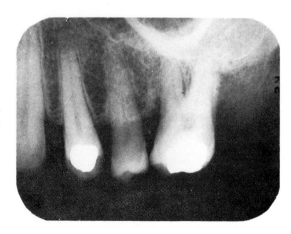

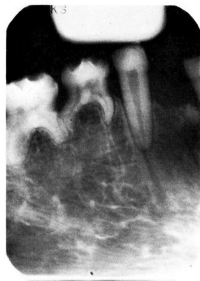

FIGURE 4-68

1. What pathologic entities can be seen in this radiograph?

2. What condition is compatible with the pathologic findings in this radiograph?

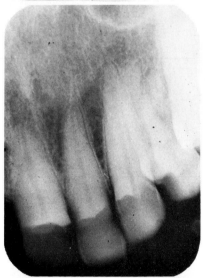

FIGURE 4-69

What change can be seen in the crowns of these teeth?

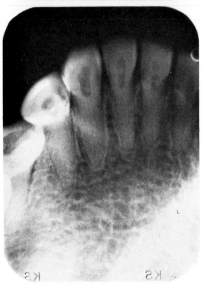

FIGURE 4-70

Janet Thistle is a 26 year old whose teeth clinically appear normal except for some attrition. Her radiograph, shown here, demonstrates the typical appearance of her condition. Her previous radiographic dental records demonstrate that her primary teeth were similarly involved. When the family history was taken, it was found that her seven year old daughter had similar involvement of both her deciduous and permanent teeth. In addition, the deciduous teeth appeared to be grayish, opalescent.

1. What radiographic changes can you observe?

2. What's the condition?

FIGURE 4–71

1. Do you think this patient has a previous history of trauma to his mandibular incisor teeth?

2. What treatment is evident in this radiograph?

3. What would you interpret this radiograph to represent?

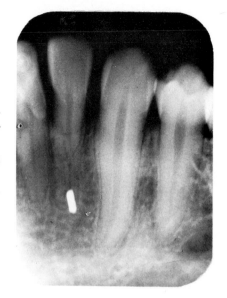

FIGURE 4–72

1. What developmental defect can be seen in association with the right deciduous central and lateral incisors?

2. What is the cause of the delayed eruption of the right permanent central and lateral incisors?

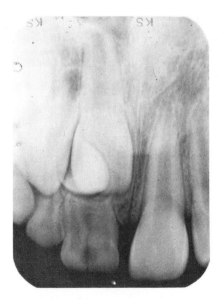

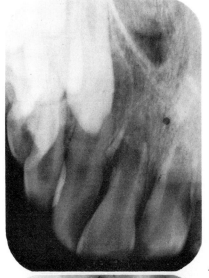

A

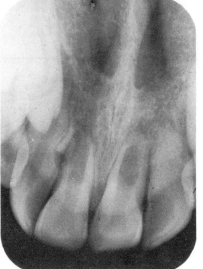

B

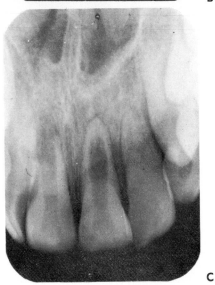

C

FIGURE 4–73

Mary Quitecontrary is a 10 year old girl who fell off her bicycle three years ago. Her teeth were sensitive and ached for a short time but eventually felt better. Recently, she has had some mild discomfort in the soft tissue high above the front teeth. Upon examination two parulides were noted in the area of the mucobuccal fold adjacent to the maxillary centrals.

What sequelae of the fall can be noted from these radiographs? Be thorough.

FIGURE 4-74

Jenny Jeans had her mandibular left second premolar extracted several years ago because of a toothache. During a recent dental visit, a Class II amalgam was placed in the mandibular left first molar. After her visit, she had sensitivity to hot and cold, and eventually a constant toothache developed. Upon reexamination it was found that the first molar was tender to percussion, and this radiograph was taken.

1. What is your diagnosis?
2. Why did this patient have pain?
3. How old is this patient?
4. What developmental anomaly is associated with the aching tooth?

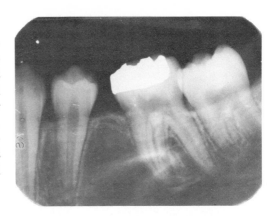

FIGURE 4-75

Identify the physiologic process that has caused these teeth to have this occlusal configuration.

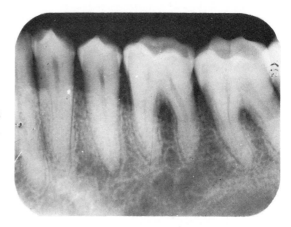

FIGURE 4-76

What developmental anomaly do you see here? Define it.

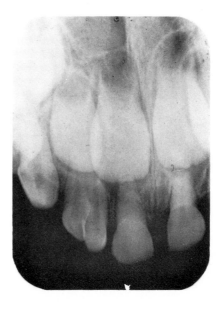

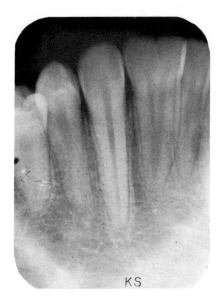

FIGURE 4–77

What developmental anomaly do you see here? Define it. (The tooth on the extreme right of the radiograph is the right central incisor.)

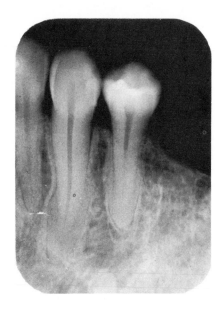

FIGURE 4–78

1. What condition is present here?
2. With what fibro-osseous lesion may this be associated?
3. Name two other conditions in which you may find this lesion.

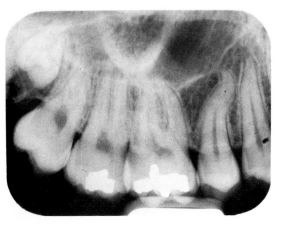

FIGURE 4–79

In viewing this radiograph, what three findings do you note? This 22 year old patient was completely asymptomatic at the time of examination. He has a previous history of chronic sinusitis.

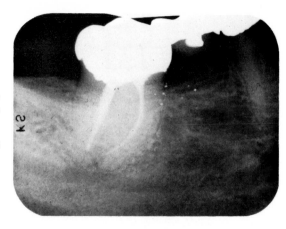

FIGURE 4–80

1. Name two good reasons why endodontic therapy was performed on this molar instead of extraction.

2. What do the little radiopaque specks at the mesial of the molar represent?

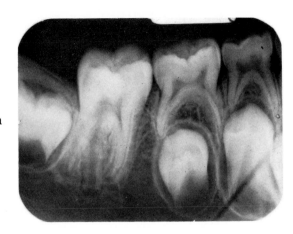

FIGURE 4–81

What developing anomaly may be seen in this radiograph?

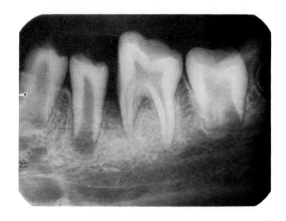

FIGURE 4–82

The features depicted in this radiograph are pathognomonic of what condition? You should know this because you've seen it before.

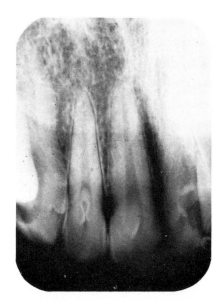

FIGURE 4–83

1. What developmental defect does this radiograph illustrate? (You've seen this before, too.)

2. Unless prevented, what is a frequent sequela?

3. How may this be prevented?

4. What tooth is most commonly affected?

5. Can this defect occur bilaterally?

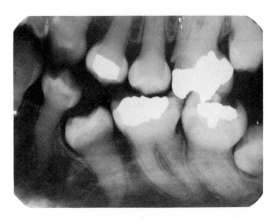

FIGURE 4–84

This should be familiar to you:

1. For what condition does this radiograph present pathognomonic evidence?

2. Is this condition hereditary?

3. Are the caries a usual finding?

4. With what other condition are the findings seen here sometimes associated?

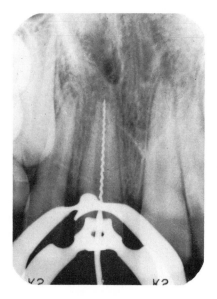

FIGURE 4–85

Is it likely that the periapical radiolucency seen in this radiograph was an indication for the endodontic procedure that is in progress? Explain your answer.

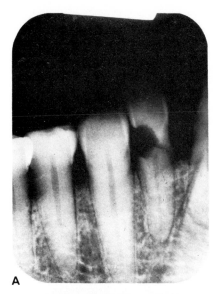

A

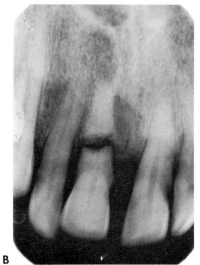

FIGURE 4–86

1. What common feature can be seen in these three radiographs?

2. Which of the three radiographs shows a pathologic condition?

3. Which of the three shows a "healed" condition?

4. Which of the three conditions has the best prognosis?

B

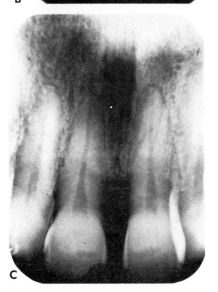

C

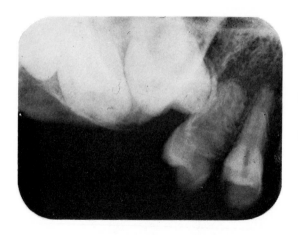

FIGURE 4–87

What unusual finding would you report upon viewing this radiograph?

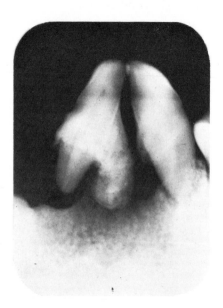

FIGURE 4–88

What is the radiopaque mass surrounding this mandibular central incisor?

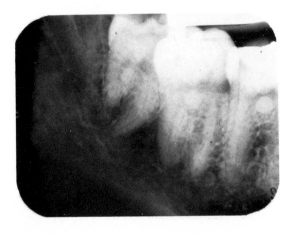

FIGURE 4–89

What are the round radiopaque structures seen close to the pulp chambers?

FIGURE 4–90

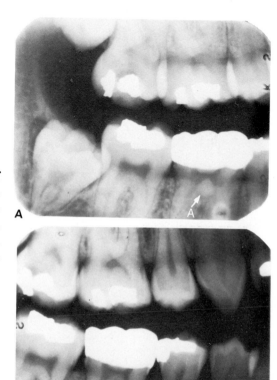

This is Mrs. Pearl Jones. She had both of these bitewing radiographs taken at the same time—i.e., with no intervening treatment between the two radiographs. Why has the "enamel pearl" at arrow A disappeared at arrow B? Now you're really going to have to do some thinking!

Lesions Affecting the Jaws

FIGURE 5-1

Mr. John Smith is 37 years old. You're looking at a routine periapical radiograph of a mandibular left molar. The patient said that the area was asymptomatic and that the mandibular left third molar was extracted approximately five years earlier.

1. Is this radiograph suggestive of a benign or a malignant lesion?

2. What is the most likely diagnosis?

3. If there were no previous history of extraction, what would be the most likely diagnosis?

4. How would you obtain a definitive diagnosis?

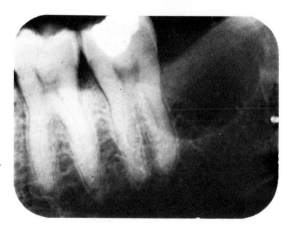

FIGURE 5-2

Marie Danielle is 13 years old and plays floor hockey, a popular Canadian school sport. She is asymptomatic. This radiolucency was discovered during a routine dental check-up. Upon questioning, she stated she was struck on the face with a hockey puck and that her jaw was quite sore for a few days.

1. With this history and radiograph, what is the most likely diagnosis?

2. What simple clinical test would be helpful in making a provisional diagnosis?

3. How would you obtain a definitive diagnosis?

4. Name four central lesions of bone that may have a similar radiographic appearance and a tendency to occur in this area.

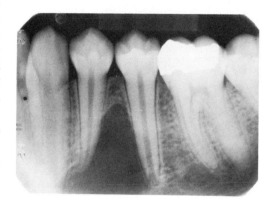

FIGURE 5-3

Sam Graingrower, a 52 year old farmer, presented to his dentist with a complaint of a tingling sensation on the left side of his lower lip. He was edentulous from the mandibular left first premolar posterior. This radiograph shows a view of the mandibular left molar area.

1. Does the lesion appear benign or malignant?

2. What is your differential diagnosis? State pros and cons for each alternative.

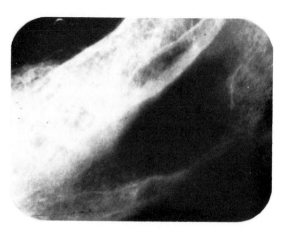

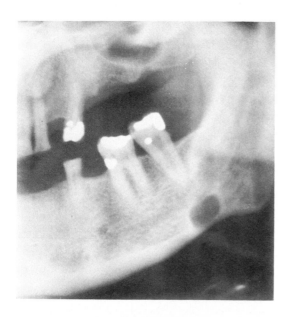

FIGURE 5–4

This asymptomatic radiolucent lesion was found upon routine examination in a 55 year old male. There was no history of trauma, and though the patient was taking diuretics for hypertension, he was otherwise healthy systemically.

1. What is this lesion?

2. Describe the radiographic features of this type of lesion.

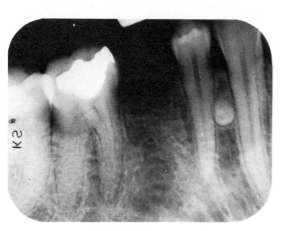

FIGURE 5–5

1. Name the two most likely explanations for the small radiopacity seen between the roots of the cuspid and first bicuspid teeth.

2. Which odontogenic cyst commonly develops in this area?

3. Name four other radiopaque entities commonly seen in this area.

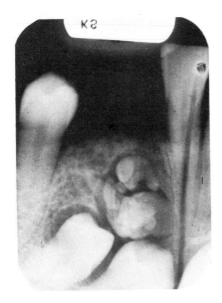

FIGURE 5–6

1. What is your interpretation of the odontogenic pathologic condition seen on this radiograph?

2. Would you send the surgical specimen in for biopsy? Give the reasons for your answer.

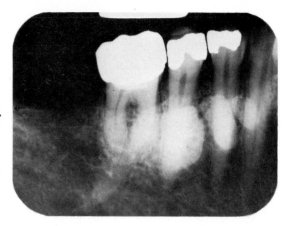

FIGURE 5–7

What would you interpret the multiple radiopacities seen in the central portion of this radiograph to represent?

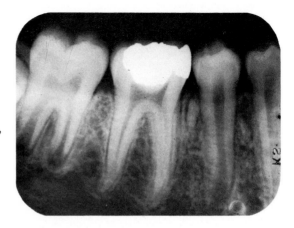

FIGURE 5–8

1. How old is this patient?
2. What pathologic entity is present?
3. Is such a lesion always iatrogenic (i.e., the result of a dental procedure)?

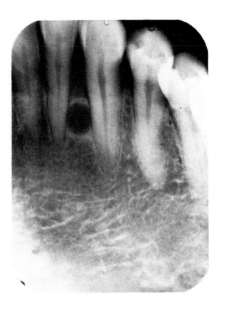

FIGURE 5–9

A lateral periodontal cyst can be seen in this radiograph.

1. State two theories concerning the etiology of such a cyst.
2. Is it possible for this cyst to have a high recurrence rate postoperatively?

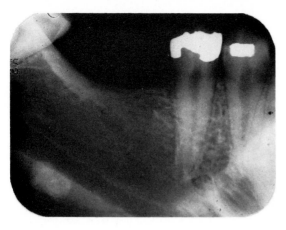

FIGURE 5–10

1. Give your differential diagnosis of the condition represented by the radiopacity at the inferior border of the mandible.

2. How would you proceed in order to obtain a more definitive radiographic diagnosis?

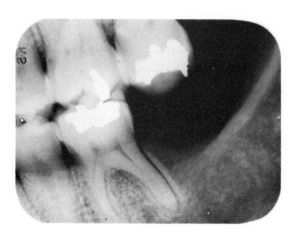

FIGURE 5–11

1. Give a differential diagnosis of a thickened periodontal membrane space.

2. Using this radiograph, substantiate your choice in this particular case. The patient is asymptomatic, and all teeth are vital.

3. Give a differential diagnosis of a thickened lamina dura.

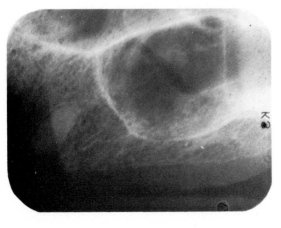

FIGURE 5–12

1. In viewing this radiograph, what finding would you report?

2. a. What is the location of this finding?

   b. What prominent radiographic landmark helps you with this location?

3. Which anatomic structure produced the well-delineated vertical line about 1 cm from the left edge of the radiograph?

FIGURE 5–13

Cherry Lee is an 18 year old female who has had this problem since age three. Clinically, her face appears swollen bilaterally; she is asymptomatic. Radiographically, bilateral multilocular expansile lesions are noted in both the mandible and maxilla.

1. What is your diagnosis?
2. Can this condition be diagnosed from radiographs alone?

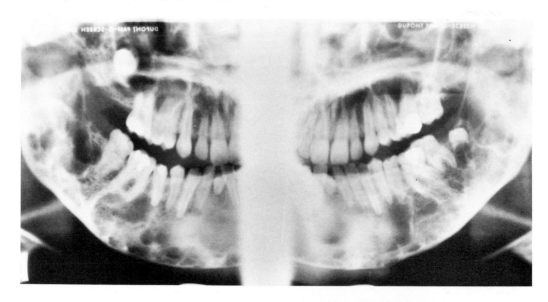

FIGURE 5–14

Comment on the trabecular pattern of the alveolar bone between the roots of the mandibular first molar.

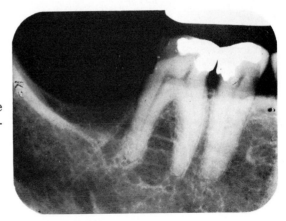

FIGURE 5–15

The patient with the three-unit bridge seen in this radiograph is a 42 year old white female. The bridge was constructed shortly after the first molar was extracted. The patient has been wearing the bridge for seven years, yet the alveolar pattern beneath the pontic does not appear normal.

1. From the radiograph, what is your diagnosis?
2. How would you confirm this?

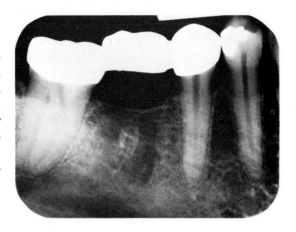

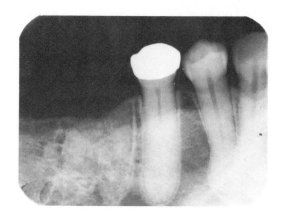

FIGURE 5–16

Cecily Glomer is 23 years old and suffers from kidney disease that has led to renal failure. For the past two years she has received dialysis treatment while awaiting a kidney transplant. About one year ago she had the lower first molar extracted.

1. When is the best time to extract a tooth of a patient on dialysis?

2. What specific lesion does the radiopaque area represent?

3. What are this lesion's characteristic radiographic features?

4. Name two broad categories of systemic disorders in which this lesion may be seen.

5. Would the mandibular second bicuspid be an easy tooth to extract?

FIGURES 5–17 THROUGH 5–23

Each of the following seven cases involves a periapical lesion. Some of the lesions are radiolucent and some are radiopaque. Some lesions are in the maxillary sinus. The purpose of this series is to help you to recognize the various presentations of inflammatory periapical lesions of pulpal origin and distinguish them from other, very similar appearing lesions that are totally unrelated to the pulp.

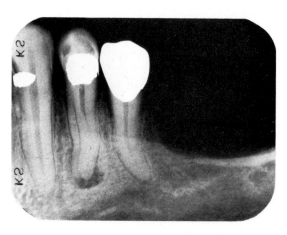

FIGURE 5–17

The mandibular first bicuspid in this radiograph is nonvital.

1. What would be your interpretation of the periapical radiolucency seen in this radiograph?

2. With what normal anatomic structures may this be confused?

3. What notable findings would you wish to pass on to the endodontist?

FIGURE 5-18

What is your interpretation of the radiopacity associated with the apex of the maxillary left second bicuspid? The tooth tested nonvital to hot, cold, and electric pulp tests.

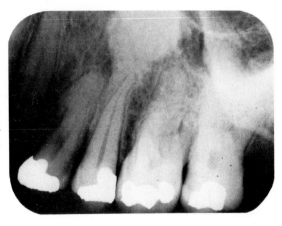

FIGURE 5-19

Give a differential diagnosis of the radiopacity at the apex of the mandibular first molar in this radiograph. The tooth is vital.

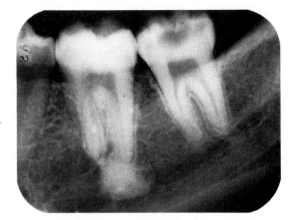

FIGURE 5-20

A 42 year old black female presented to the clinic for a recall examination. The routine periapical radiograph revealed multiple radiolucencies about the apices of the mandibular anterior teeth. The teeth were asymptomatic, tested vital, and were not sensitive to percussion.

1. What is your diagnosis and recommended treatment?

2. What condition is this said to closely resemble?

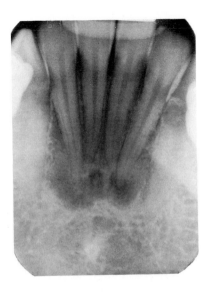

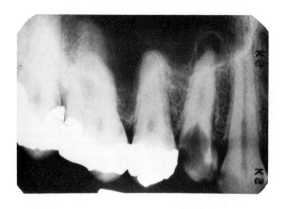

FIGURE 5–21

Give a differential diagnosis of the radiolucency at the apex of the maxillary right first bicuspid.

By now you should know this cold.

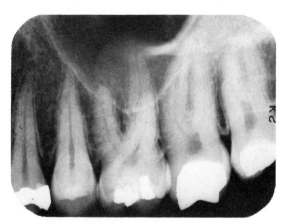

FIGURE 5–22

All of the maxillary teeth are vital to pulp tests.

1. What radiopaque lesion may be seen in the maxillary sinus?

2. An identical lesion may be seen in another condition—one associated with pulp inflammation. What is this other condition?

3. Why is the distinction between the two conditions important?

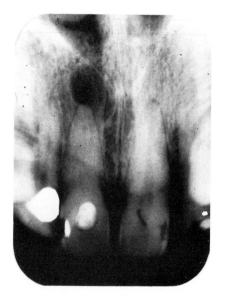

FIGURE 5–23

1. Give a differential diagnosis of the large periapical lesion seen in this radiograph. Keep in mind the anatomic location of this lesion.

2. In the absence of an adequate history and on the basis of this radiograph what, do you suppose, led to the development of this lesion?

FIGURE 5–24

1. What is your differential diagnosis of the lesion in the left maxilla?

2. What is the cause of the large radiolucent area affecting most of the maxilla?

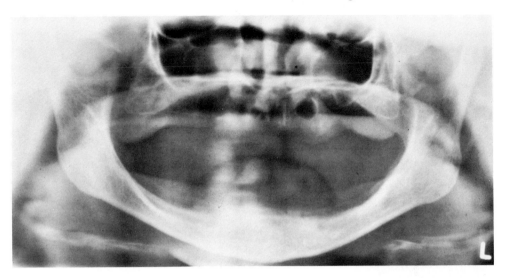

FIGURE 5–25

George Lovejoy is a 19 year old college student who attended his older sister's wedding reception two days before his problem began. Thanks to a copious flow of pink champagne, George was feeling no pain but vaguely remembers hitting himself in the face with the refrigerator door in response to an urgent request for more ice cubes. His chief complaint was that his jaw "hurt" when he masticated food. The third molar was vital.

What is your diagnosis?

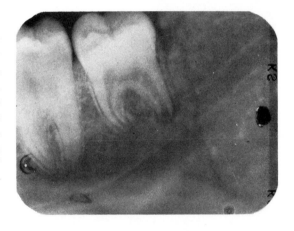

FIGURE 5–26

The patient had a toothache some time ago but is currently asymptomatic.

1. Identify the radiolucent area at arrow A.

2. Interpret the radiographic findings in association with the following areas of the maxillary second bicuspid:

    a. coronal portion,

    b. root, and

    c. periapical region.

Be careful! You should get this.

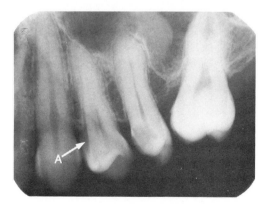

FIGURE 5–27

This case involves a 20 year old male patient who presented with a large swelling on the right side of the face. He stated that the swelling was present for several years, but he never sought treatment. All teeth were vital and there were no skin lesions or other bony defects.

1. Give a differential diagnosis of this lesion.

2. What do you think this lesion is?

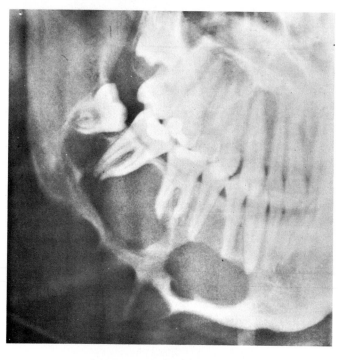

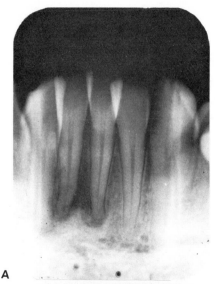

A

FIGURE 5–28

Three different patients' radiographs are shown in *A*, *B*, and *C*. All three patients have the same condition and are typical of most patients with this condition.

1. Are these patients black or white?
2. How old are these patients?
3. Are they male or female?
4. Are these teeth likely to be vital?
5. What is the name of the condition?

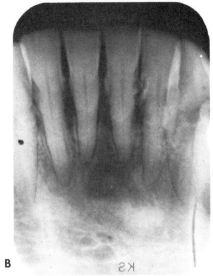

B

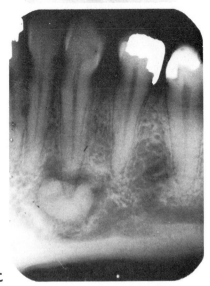

C

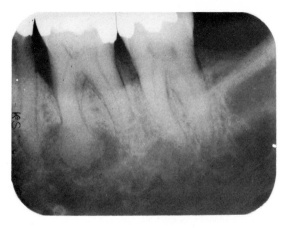

FIGURE 5-29

1. What is your impression of the radiopacity associated with the mesial root of the mandibular first molar?

2. Is this the common location for this lesion?

3. What is the treatment? Give the reasons for your answer.

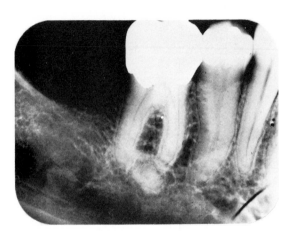

FIGURE 5-30

This radiograph was part of a routine full-mouth survey of a 43 year old black female. A small hole in the occlusal of the crown, prepared without the aid of anesthesia, revealed that the mandibular first molar was vital. The patient was asymptomatic.

What is your impression of the radiopacity at the apex of the first molar? (Clinically the lesion was well delineated by a radiolucent area that extended to and included the apex of the distal root.)

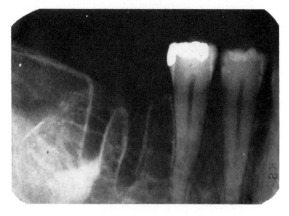

FIGURE 5-31

With the help of this radiograph, explain the reason for the extraction of the mandibular first molar.

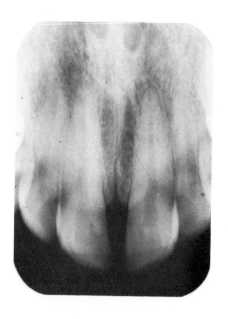

FIGURE 5–32

What developmental defect may be visualized here? Let's see how good you are.

FIGURE 5–33

1. What developmental defect of the jaws do you see?

2. What other developmental defect is present?

3. What structure does the oval-shaped radiopacity in the middle of the defect represent?

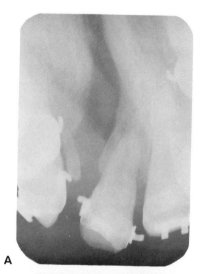

A

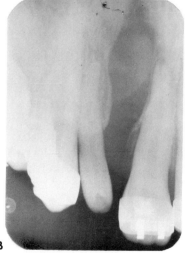

B

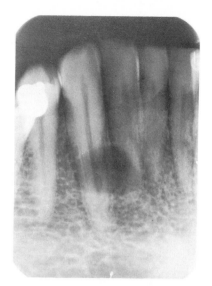

FIGURE 5–34

The patient, a 46 year old male, was asymptomatic. Upon examination a palpable depression was noted on the lingual aspect of the mandible level with the floor of the mouth in the cuspid area. This area was not tender, and all teeth were vital. There was no history of trauma. What developmental condition does this radiolucent area represent?

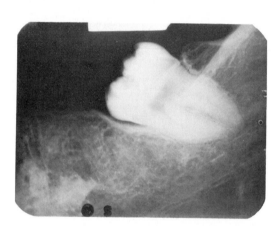

FIGURE 5–35

What anatomic variation can be seen in this radiograph?

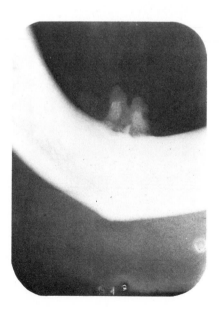

FIGURE 5–36

1. What anatomic variation is seen here?
2. Is this of any clinical significance?

FIGURE 5–37

Dental care in this case was sought by a 19 year old patient who had several episodes of acute pain on various occasions. The panoramic film revealed a pericoronal radiolucency in the left mandibular molar–ramus area.

1. What panoramic patient positioning error was made in taking this film?

2. What caused the radiolucency across the apices of most of the maxillary teeth?

3. Give a differential diagnosis of the lesion in the left mandible.

4. What is the most likely diagnosis?

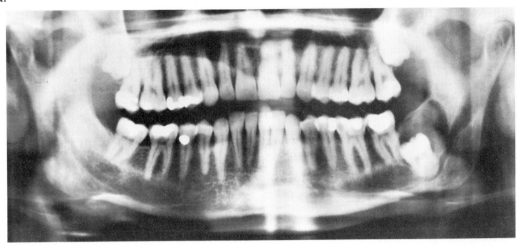

FIGURE 5–38

This case involves a 55 year old female patient who has been edentulous for about 5 years. Recently her dentures became loose and she came to the dentist to have new ones fitted. She was asymptomatic and this film was taken as part of the routine examination.

1. List the possible diagnoses you may make regarding the lesion in the midline of the maxilla.

2. Which should be your choice for the most likely diagnosis?

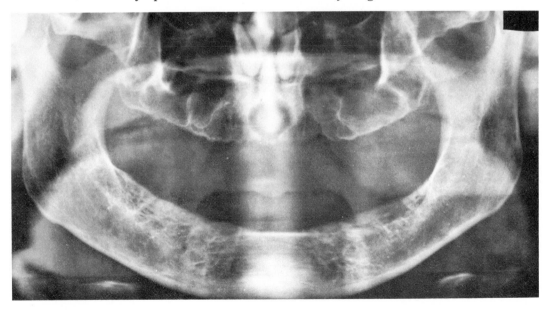

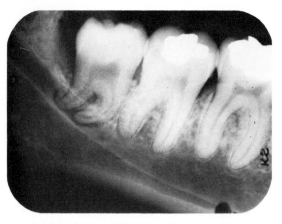

FIGURE 5–39

This radiograph was difficult to take because the patient, a 19 year old male, exhibited trismus and some sensitivity in the molar area. Additional symptoms with which the patient presented included swelling of the right side of the face, low-grade fever, and earache.

1. What is your diagnosis?
2. Will the third molar erupt any further? Give the reason for your answer.

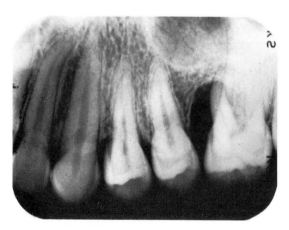

FIGURE 5–40

The patient in this case, a 19 year old black female, had absolutely perfect dentition upon visual inspection. The soft tissue appeared normal, and the patient was asymptomatic. The routine radiographs showed almost identical lesions in all four quadrants. The oral hygiene was adequate.

1. Give a differential diagnosis.
2. What is the most likely diagnosis?

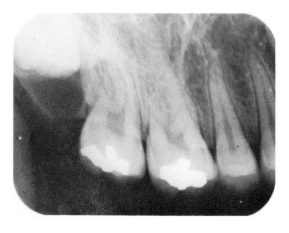

FIGURE 5–41

Johnny Every is 21 years old and is having slight discomfort in the posterior portion of his mouth. Upon examination, you notice that the gingiva on the crest of the ridge distal to the second molar appears swollen and slightly bluish in color. This radiograph was taken at the time of examination. No treatment was given. The patient was asymptomatic within 15 days.

What is your diagnosis?

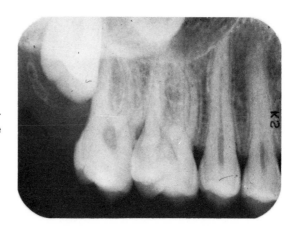

FIGURE 5–42

What is your diagnosis of the small radiopacity associated with the crown of the erupting third molar?

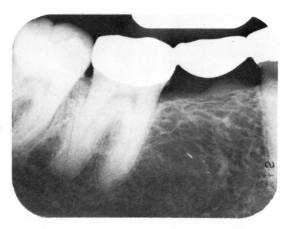

FIGURE 5–43

What term is used to describe the radiopaque bump on the alveolar ridge under the pontic?

FIGURE 5–44

These radiographs are from two different patients, both of whom are female, in their mid-forties, asymptomatic, and healthy.

What lesion do both patients have?

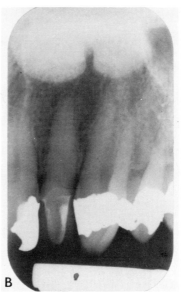

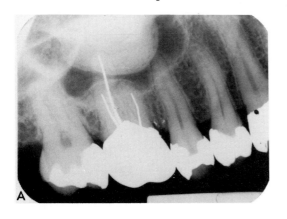

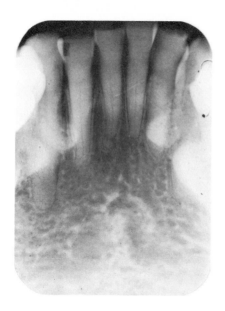

FIGURE 5–45

Name at least five separate findings that you should report from your observation of this radiograph.

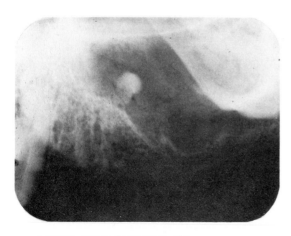

FIGURE 5–46

Give a differential diagnosis of the small circular radiopaque structure seen in association with the maxillary sinus.

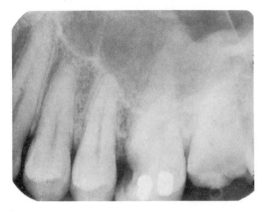

FIGURE 5–47

Approximately 80 per cent of the maxillary sinus in this radiograph appears somewhat opaque, whereas the remainder appears radiolucent. In viewing this radiograph, how would you interpret these findings?

All of the next lesions have similarities and it may be helpful to study them as a group.

FIGURE 5–48

Here is a situation in which two patients have the same lesion but at different stages. The mature lesion is pathognomonic. The male patient is asymptomatic, as is the female patient. In fact, both patients are in their mid-twenties, and in both cases the mandibular molars are vital, are free of caries, and have never been restored.

1. Which is the mature lesion?
2. What radiographic similarities and differences are there between the lesion at the stage shown in A and that at the stage shown in B?
3. What is the diagnosis?
4. What treatment is required?

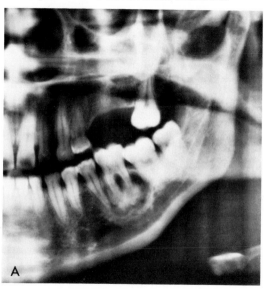

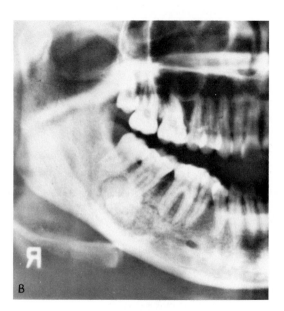

FIGURE 5–49

This radiograph was taken upon routine examination of a 19 year old female patient of Mexican-American extraction. She has never had orthodontic treatment. The mandibular second premolar is vital. The patient has no systemic problems, and there is no history of intestinal polyps.

1. What lesion do you think is present? (*Hint:* You've seen this before!)
2. Comment upon the length of the bicuspid roots.

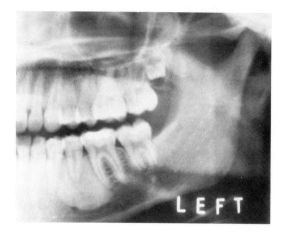

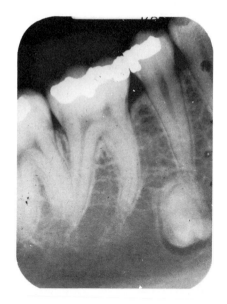

FIGURE 5–50

1. What is your diagnosis of this radiopaque lesion?

2. Are the radiographic findings sufficient to warrant surgical excision?

3. Is the radiographic picture sufficient for use in establishing the final diagnosis of the case? Give the reasons for your answer.

FIGURE 5–51

The radiograph shows a lesion found in a 34 year old white male who was seen mainly for a complaint of intermittent sensitivity to hot and cold in the mandibular left molar region. The large restorations in the area were present for years. Examination revealed expansion of the buccal and lingual cortical plates in the region of the left bicuspid molar area. All of the teeth were vital.

1. Give a differential diagnosis of the lesion in the left mandible.

2. What diagnostic possibility is the best choice?

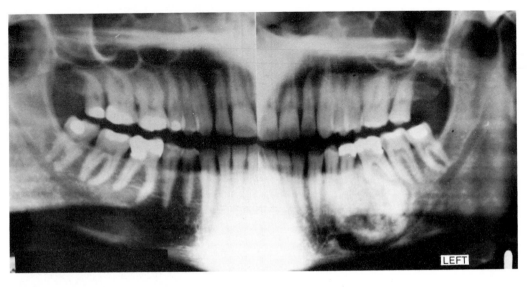

FIGURE 5–52

The patient, a 32 year old white male, presented with mild paresthesia in the lower lip on the left side. He knew that he had some impacted "wisdom" teeth and came in to see if this was the cause. Upon examination there was no evidence of expansion in the left side of the mandible, and the overlying soft tissue appeared normal. Give a differential diagnosis of the lesion in the left mandible.

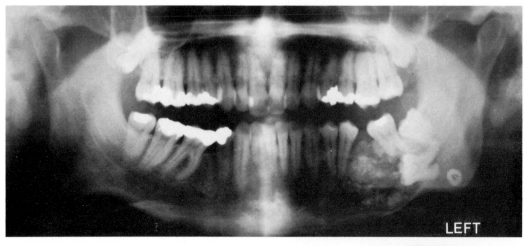

FIGURE 5–53

The patient is a 19 year old male with an asymptomatic mild swelling in the right side of his face. What do you think this lesion is? (*Hint:* This lesion is often associated with one or more impacted or unerupted teeth, occurs during the tooth-forming years of life, and is histologically characterized by the presence of enamel matrix.)

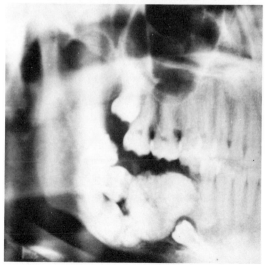

FIGURE 5–54

What lesion is present in the maxillary sinus?

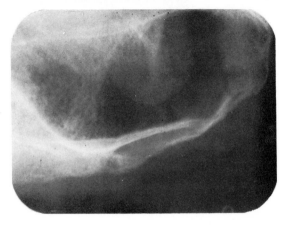

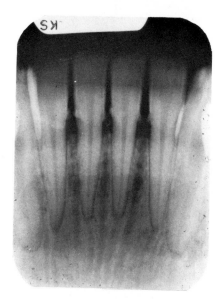

FIGURE 5–55

1. What anatomic structure do the radiolucent vertical lines represent?

2. What is the radiopaque material in the cervical area of these teeth?

3. With what disease may the two preceding entities be associated?

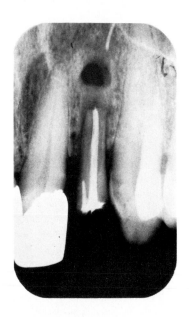

FIGURE 5–56

This case involves a patient with a history of an apicoectomy of the maxillary lateral incisor. What condition does the radiolucency in this radiograph represent?

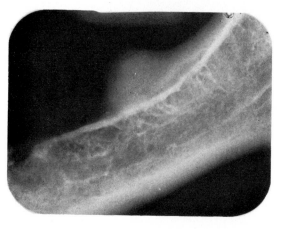

FIGURE 5–57

A biopsy of this asymptomatic lesion on the crest of the mandibular edentulous ridge revealed normal lamellar bone. What is your diagnosis and treatment?

FIGURE 5–58

A 26 year old white female presented to the clinic for a routine examination. The periapical radiograph of the mandibular left molar region is shown. The teeth were asymptomatic and tested vital, and the serum calcium level proved to be 9 mg per 100 ml.

1. Describe the radiographic appearance of this lesion.

2. Prior to obtaining lab results, what is your differential diagnosis?

3. If all other lab values were normal, what would be your tentative diagnosis prior to biopsy?

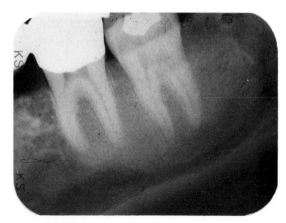

FIGURE 5–59

Lisa Glomer is 24 years old and, like her sister, has renal problems. Specifically, Lisa has chronic glomerulonephritis. Although her blood is being dialyzed regularly, it has averaged the following values: 12.5 mg of Ca per 100 ml; 1.6 mg of inorganic phosphate per 100 ml; 15 King-Armstrong units of alkaline phosphatase per 100 ml. Histologically, the lesion that was resorbing the molar roots contained giant cells. Urinary excretion of Ca on a low-calcium diet was 203 mg per liter. She had metastatic calcification in some of her fingers, as well as in other areas. What was her systemic condition that produced the changes seen in these two radiographs?

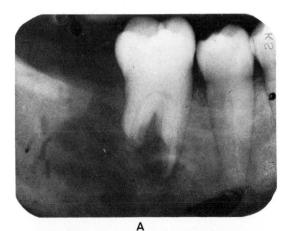

A

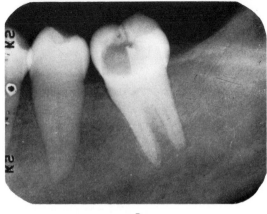

B

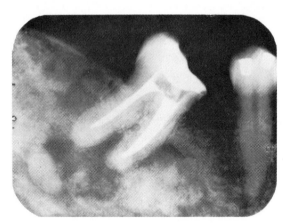

FIGURE 5–60

This case involves a 57 year old male patient with a history of pain in the weight-bearing joints. The alkaline phosphatase level is 156 Bodansky units. He has had several complete maxillary dentures constructed, each one becoming too tight after some years' use.

1. With the aid of the radiograph, tell what condition this history suggests.

2. What radiographic features of this condition can be seen here?

3. Radiographic findings closely resembling those presented here may be noted in what other condition?

FIGURE 5–61

The radiograph shows multiple radiopaque masses throughout the mandible in a 48 year old black female. The patient was asymptomatic and was not aware of her condition. There was a history of multiple fistulas and sequestration of bone.

1. Give a differential diagnosis.

2. What is the patient's condition?

3. What treatment would you prescribe?

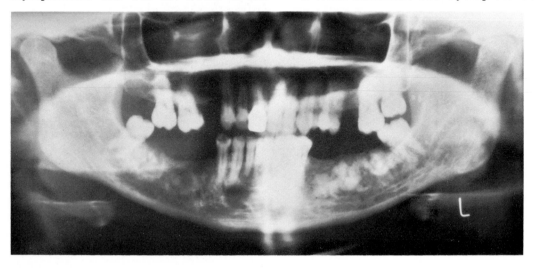

FIGURE 5–62

The patient, a 26 year old white female, presented with pain in the left mandible and a history of recent weight loss. The pain had developed after routine extraction of the mandibular left third molar and had been unsuccessfully treated for a six-week period with various local dressings in the extraction socket. The patient's husband stated that she had lost 15 pounds and that he frankly suspected that she may have cancer.

Upon examination, several tender lymph nodes were palpable in the left submaxillary area. The extraction socket appeared to contain no clot or granulation tissue. The mandibular left first and second bicuspids were extremely mobile and tested nonvital with the electric pulp test. A fistulous tract could be traced from the lingual of the first molar to an area between the apices of the first and second bicuspids. Radiographically, the trabecular pattern had markedly changed from the normal pattern seen one year earlier (Fig. A).

Pulp biopsies of the mandibular first and second bicuspids revealed normal viable pulps. A high-protein diet and antibiotics were prescribed. The patient gradually improved, and penicillin treatment was discontinued after six weeks. Endodontic therapy was completed on the mandibular first and second bicuspids.

What's your diagnosis?

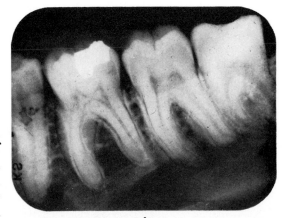

A

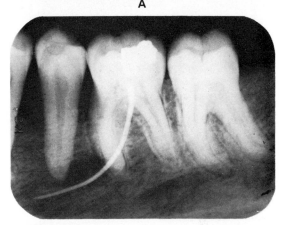

B

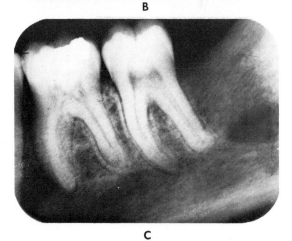

C

FIGURE 5–63

This case involves a 9 year old who first presented with swelling in the right side of the face and a low grade fever. A deeply carious mandibular right first molar was discovered and extracted. One week later the child returned because his face was still swollen and a low grade fever of 100°F was still present. Intraorally there was a bone-hard swelling buccal to the extraction site, the overlying tissue was slightly red, and the depth of the mucobuccal fold was markedly diminished in the area. This radiograph was taken at the second visit. The bone appeared different in the right body of the mandible. Additionally, a distinct periosteal reaction could be seen at the inferior border of the right mandible, and several layers of subperiosteal new bone were visible.

1. Give a differential diagnosis.
2. What is your diagnosis?
3. How would you treat this?

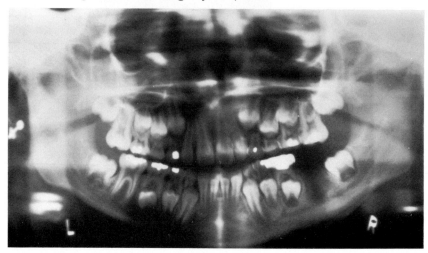

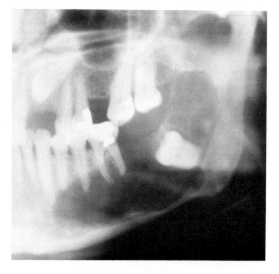

FIGURE 5–64

This lesion was found on routine examination of an asymptomatic 35 year old male. The biopsy proved the lesion to be an *odontogenic keratocyst* (OKC).

1. What sub-type of OKC is this?
2. Can you name the other sub-types?
3. What are the radiographic features of the OKC?
4. With what syndrome is the OKC sometimes associated? Describe the salient features of this syndrome.
5. What is so important about distinguishing OKC's from other odontogenic, fissural, and developmental cysts?

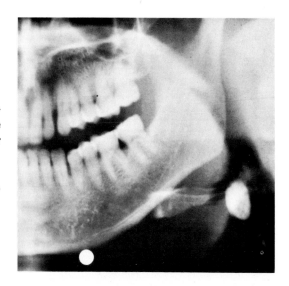

FIGURE 5–65

Below the angle of the mandible two separate radiopaque entities may be seen. One is a normal anatomic structure; the other represents a pathologic finding.

  1. Identify the normal structure.

  2. Give a differential diagnosis of the abnormality.

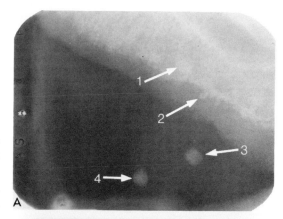

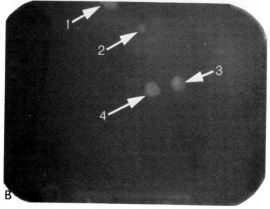

FIGURE 5–66

The patient is a 65 year old edentulous male with no particular complaint except that he wished to have new dentures made. The four calcifications seen in radiograph A were determined to be in the buccal mucosa by taking radiograph B.

  1. How was radiograph B taken? Include film placement and relative exposure values as compared to what may have been used in A.

  2. Give a differential diagnosis for the four radiopacities seen.

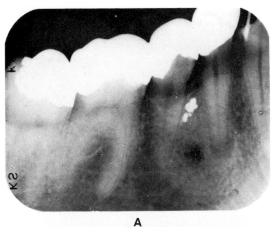

A

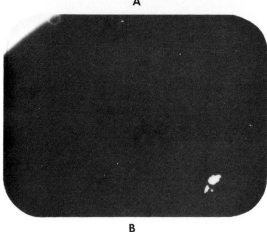

B

FIGURE 5–67

The patient was a 27 year old woman who was no stranger to dental treatment. When the radiopacity between the two bicuspids was noted, the area was checked clinically for the presence of an amalgam tattoo on the alveolar mucosa. No such lesion was seen. Where do you suppose the amalgam tattoo was finally located?

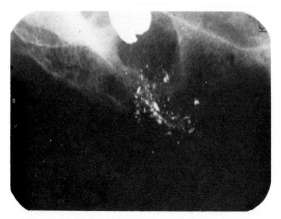

FIGURE 5–68

Give a differential diagnosis of the radiopaque material seen in this radiograph.

FIGURE 5–69

This case involves a 70 year old female patient who came in for new prostheses. The patient was not in pain, had no known systemic disorders, and had never broken any bones.

1. What are the bilateral radiopacities at arrows A?

2. What patient positioning error caused these to be superimposed upon the mandible?

3. What is the cause of the radiolucent shadow crossing both sides of the maxilla?

4. Now look carefully at all of the bone. Disregard the radiolucent panoramic artifact in the anterior midline of the mandible. Do you see that there is very little cortical bone and that the remainder of the bone does not appear very radiopaque? What bone disorder does this elderly female patient have?

5. How is this disorder treated?

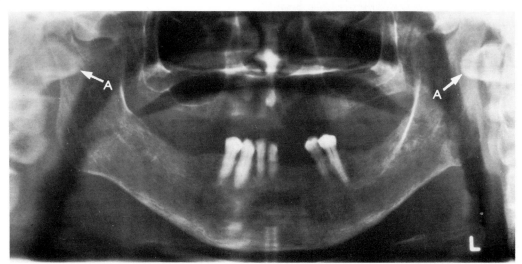

FIGURE 5–70

The radiograph shows a lesion found in a 22 year old female patient who had presented for a routine examination. She had no pain and she could remember no recent trauma. She had no constitutional symptoms. Aspiration yielded a slight bit of blood. Findings on biopsy prompted follow-up examinations for evaluation of the patient's serum calcium levels. The levels were found to be normal, and averaged 10.5 mg/dl over three readings on three separate days.

1. Based upon the radiograph, give a differential diagnosis.

2. Based upon the history, what is the diagnosis?

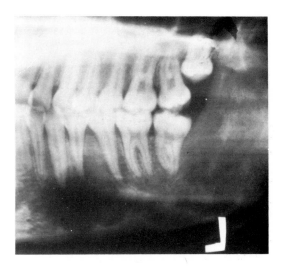

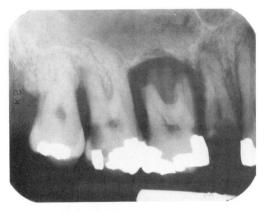

FIGURE 5–71

The patient in this case is a 35 year old male who has poor oral hygiene, drinks heavily, and smokes a lot. He came in to have a loose tooth extracted. This radiograph was taken and a "floating tooth" was discovered. What is the differential diagnosis in this situation.

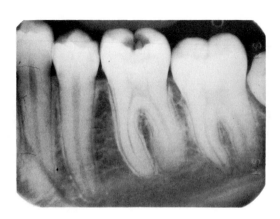

FIGURE 5–72

A 12 year old male presented to the clinic complaining of sensitivity to hot, cold, and sweets in the mandibular left posterior region. After a sedative dressing had been in place for three months, all teeth tested vital.

Based on these findings, what is your recommended diagnosis and treatment?

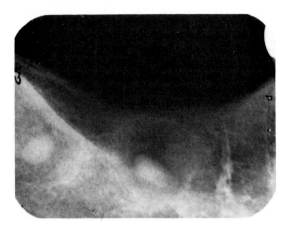

FIGURE 5–73

This is a periapical radiograph taken as part of a routine full-mouth radiographic survey of a 46 year old black edentulous female. She is currently asymptomatic.

1. Which anatomic area is shown on this radiograph?

2. Give a differential diagnosis of the lesions seen.

3. Which alternative is your most likely choice?

FIGURE 5–74

A 35 year old edentulous male presented to the clinic for a routine examination prior to having a new complete maxillary denture constructed.

1. Of what region is this radiograph?
2. Which tooth is this?
3. What would be your most likely diagnosis of the condition represented by the radiolucency about the crown of the unerupted tooth?
4. Which odontogenic tumor, often associated with an impacted tooth, frequently occurs in this area?
5. What is the large radiolucency superior to the root portion of this tooth?

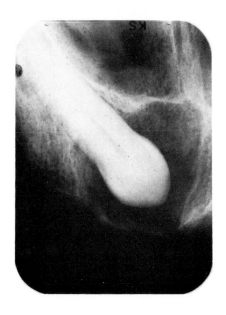

FIGURE 5–75

What types of odontomas are indicated by the morphological features visualized in these radiographs?

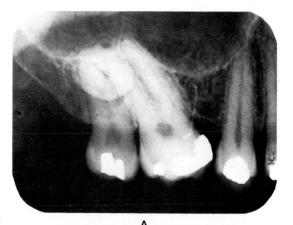

A

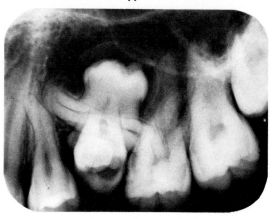

B

Localization Techniques

LOCALIZATION OF OBJECTS OR STRUCTURES

The Buccal Object Rule

It is sometimes necessary to determine whether foreign objects or dental structures are buccally or lingually situated. A relatively easy method for doing this is called the buccal object rule or shift. It is necessary to take two separate radiographs of the area in question. The first radiograph is taken using the proper intra-oral technique. The second radiograph is taken by changing the position of the x-ray cone. The flow of the x-ray beam is directed toward either the anterior or the posterior. If the object or structure is located buccally, it will appear to have shifted in the direction that the radiographic beam is flowing. If the object or structure is located lingually or palatally, it will appear to have moved toward the source of radiation. Refer to the diagrams.

Diagram 1A is an occlusal view in the mandibular premolar-molar area. The dark object is located on the buccal surface, and we can see it in that position.

The periapical view in Diagram 1B is the same area shown in 1A. In order to demonstrate the position of the foreign object, merely take a second periapical like the one in Diagram 1C. The radiation flows from the posterior to the anterior. Note that the object has moved toward the anterior. This indicates that it is located buccally.

Now, take a look at Diagram 2A. The dark round objects are located at the apices of the premolars. When the second radiograph is taken as shown in Diagram 2B, the most anterior object moves more toward the anterior. You must realize that the direction of radiation flow is from the posterior to the anterior. The anterior object is thus a buccal object, and the other object is most likely attached to the apex of the second premolar. Well, that's all the explanation you need.

Now that you understand this principle, try the following exercises:

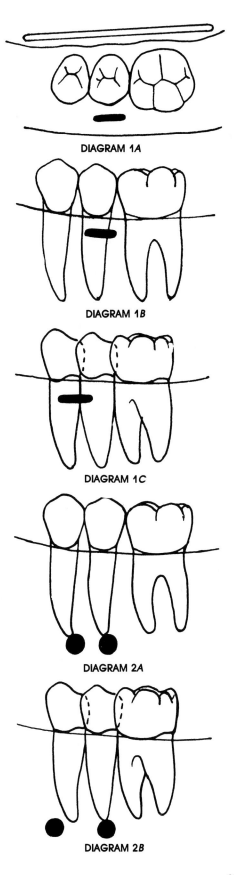

DIAGRAM 1A

DIAGRAM 1B

DIAGRAM 1C

DIAGRAM 2A

DIAGRAM 2B

FIGURE 6-1

1. What is the radiopaque structure located at the tip of the arrow in Figure 6–1A called?

2. In Figure 6–1B it appears to have shifted its position distally. Is it located palatally or buccally?

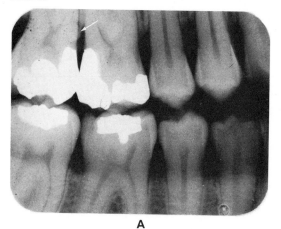

A

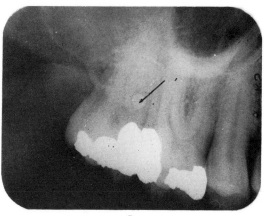

B

FIGURE 6-2

Where is the impacted third molar located in relation to the second molar? Figure 6–2A was taken in the usual, prescribed manner, whereas Figure 6–2B was taken with the x-ray cone directed toward the anterior of the arch.

What's your answer? Remember the rule.

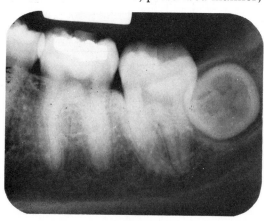

A

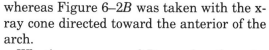

B

FIGURE 6–3

If you look closely at Figure 6–3A, you won't see anything unusual in the root structure of the first molar. In Figure 6–3B the horizontal angulation of the x-ray cone was changed so that the beam flow was toward the anterior of the arch. What do you see in this radiograph? Is it located buccally or lingually?

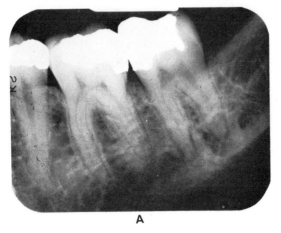

A

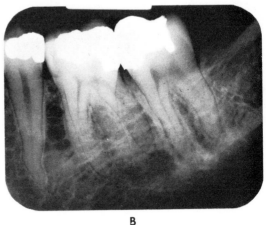

B

FIGURE 6–4

The buccal object rule works not only on the horizontal plane but also on the vertical plane. Here's a good example. The arrow in Figure 6–4A is pointing to a small silver alloy. This radiograph was taken using a negative vertical angulation, whereas Figure 6–4B was taken using a positive vertical angulation. Note how the small silver alloy separated from the occlusal silver alloy in the latter radiograph. Is this small silver alloy located buccally or lingually?

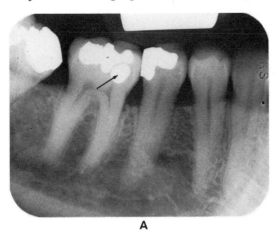

A

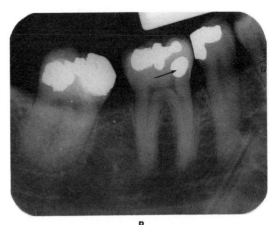

B

FIGURE 6–5

This is another example of the buccal object rule used in the vertical plane. Figure 6–5A was taken at a positive vertical angulation, whereas Figure 6–5B was taken at a much higher positive vertical angulation. The arrow in Figure 6–5B indicates that the small silver alloy is moving or shifting up instead of down. It is moving toward the source of radiation and not in the same direction as the beam flow. Is this small silver alloy located buccally or lingually?

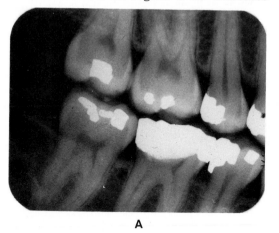

A

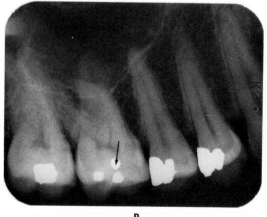

B

FIGURE 6–6

In Figure 6–6A, there is a radiopaque image located over the mesial proximal root surface of the second bicuspid. Figure 6–6B was taken with a horizontal change of the x-ray cone. The x-ray beam was directed anteriorly. Note the change of the radiopaque image. It is now slightly distal to the mesial root surface of the second bicuspid. Is it located lingually or buccally?

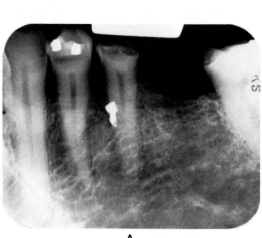

A

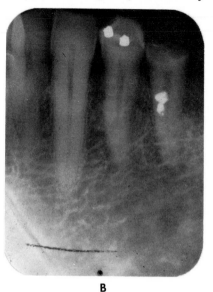

B

Panoramic Localization

Panoramic localization may be done only in some situations, usually in the anterior region. There are two methods, one using the "SLOB" rule with the split image and the other using *"object magnification"* in any image. We will first cover how the SLOB rule works. Suppose you have a patient with an impacted canine, and because of the chair shift you see two images of it, as in Figure 6–7. The acronym SLOB means **S**ame on **L**ingual, **O**pposite on **B**uccal. The beauty of this extremely simple technique is that you need not worry how the film was exposed, or which way the machine moved. You simply look at the two images of the object in the radiograph. In Figure 6–7 look at the tip of the crown on the patient's left side: it is superimposed on the left central incisor. Now shift your gaze toward the patient's right side. The question you must now answer is: *did the tooth move in the same direction as my gaze or in the opposite direction?* If the tooth moves in the same direction as one's gaze, the tooth will be seen more toward the patient's right and it will be on the lingual. If the tooth moves in the opposite direction of one's gaze, it will be more toward the patient's left and therefore be located on the buccal. Remember, *Same on Lingual, Opposite on Buccal.* Now you're ready to try Figure 6–7.

FIGURE 6–7

We took a skull and taped an extracted tooth to it, and then took this panoramic film. The question: did we tape the tooth onto the palate, or onto the buccal plate?

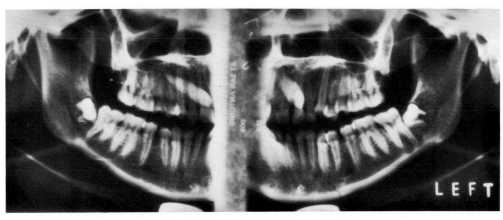

FIGURE 6–8

Now this is a real case. It was discovered that the patient, a young man, was shot with a B-B gun sometime during his child- hood. Where would you look for the B-B? In the lip, or somewhere behind the teeth? (By the way, the teeth were sound and vital.)

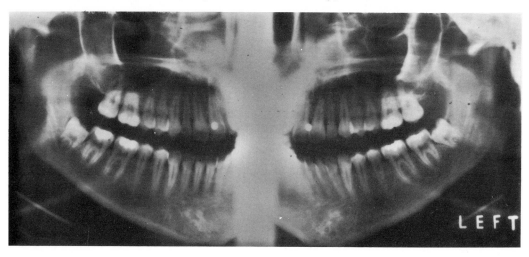

Another method of localization with panoramic films involves the use of the panoramic principle of *"object magnification."* As we saw in the patient positioning errors, the teeth become too slim if the patient is too far forward in the machine and too fat if the patient is positioned too far back. It follows then that objects toward the buccal of the focal trough will be slimmer than those in the center, and objects on the lingual side of the focal trough will be wider. Now, go to Figure 6–9 and try this out.

FIGURE 6–9

In studying this panoramic film, you note an impacted right cuspid. If this tooth were to be extracted or surgically ligated for or- thodontic traction it would be important to know whether this tooth is located more toward the palate or more toward the buccal. What is the tooth's location?

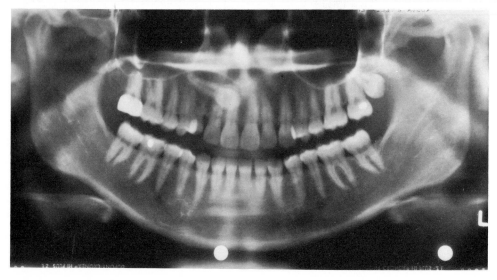

section 7

Review Questions for National and State Board Examinations

FIGURE 7–1

Select the most appropriate term for the anomaly to which the arrow is pointing.
A. Diastema
B. Concrescence
C. Dilaceration
D. Dens invaginatus

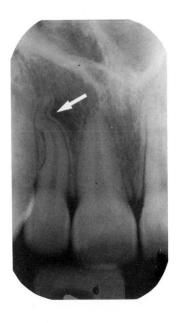

FIGURE 7–2

The patient is a 60 year old male with markedly shortened crowns. He does not smoke a pipe; nor does he work in an environment where particulate matter or acid-containing fumes can pollute the air. He has no known eating disorders and is systemically healthy.

By what process have the crowns acquired this appearance?
A. Attrition
B. Abrasion
C. Erosion
D. Amelogenesis imperfecta

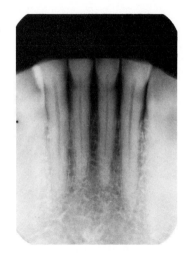

FIGURE 7–3

To what developmental anomaly is the arrow pointing?
A. Phlebolith
B. Cementoma
C. Dentinoma
D. Enameloma

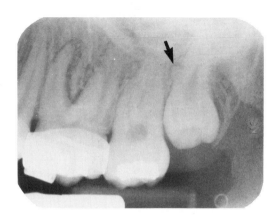

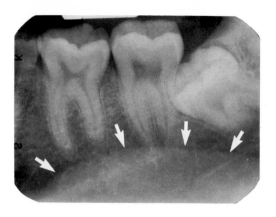

FIGURE 7–4

The arrows are pointing to a radiopaque area at the apices of the mandibular molars. Both of the erupted molars are vital, and no hard bony mass or expansion could be found on the buccal or lingual cortical plates.

Select the most appropriate cause of this radiopacity.

A. Osteosclerosis
B. Osteoma
C. Benign cementoblastoma
D. Tongue shadow

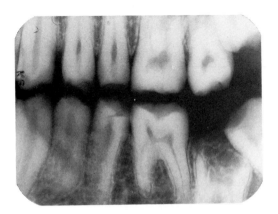

FIGURE 7–5

Yellower than normal clinically, the teeth shown here have had this radiographic appearance ever since they erupted; the primary teeth of the patient, a 25 year old male, looked just like this as well. The patient does not suffer from bulimia or anorexia nervosa, nor has he ever had much of a problem with caries.

What condition affects these teeth?

A. Erosion
B. Amelogenesis imperfecta
C. Dentinogenesis imperfecta
D. Attrition

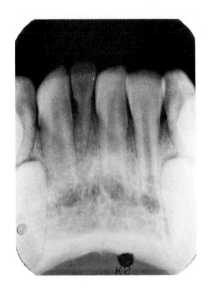

FIGURE 7–6

All of the teeth seen in this radiograph are vital.

1. What important condition should be ruled out in association with the congenitally missing mandibular central incisor?

    A. Cleidocranial dysplasia
    B. Ectodermal dysplasia
    C. Rieger's syndrome
    D. Incontinentia pigmenti

2. The multiple periapical radiolucencies in this radiograph are due to:

    A. Periapical abscess, granuloma, or cyst
    B. Dental papilla
    C. Periapical cemental dysplasia
    D. Chronic osteomyelitis

FIGURE 7–7

In this radiograph, multiple pulp stones are present. Although they are usually of no significance, they are important in:

A. The diagnosis of dentin dysplasia, type I

B. The diagnosis of dentin dysplasia, type II

C. Endodontic treatment planning

D. All of the above

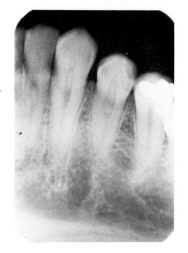

FIGURE 7–8

In this radiograph all of the teeth are vital. The patient is asymptomatic, and no abnormality could be detected clinically.

1. What term *best* describes the space at arrow A?

    A. Diastema

    B. Dilaceration

    C. Primate space

    D. None of the above

2. What is the cause of the radiolucency at arrow B?

    A. Lateral fossa

    B. Lateral periodontal cyst

    C. Globulomaxillary cyst

    D. Adenomatoid odontogenic tumor

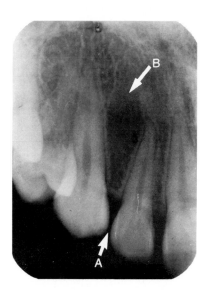

FIGURE 7–9

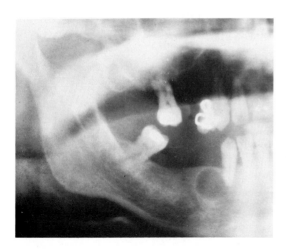

The lesion in the right body of the mandible was removed and the pathologist reported that it was a lateral periodontal cyst. From the list below select the most appropriate statement concerning this lesion.

A. As the pathologist reported, it is a lateral periodontal cyst, and no more information is needed.

B. It is a lateral periodontal cyst, but I need to know if it is an odontogenic keratocyst subtype.

C. It is a lateral periodontal cyst, and it can't be an odontogenic keratocyst.

D. The lesion is a lateral periodontal cyst, and it would be interesting to know if the cyst is an odontogenic keratocyst subtype—although there's no significant difference between the two.

FIGURE 7–10

Please answer the following questions relating to this panoramic film.

1. What patient positioning error occurred in the taking of this film?
   A. Patient too far forward
   B. Patient too far back
   C. Chin tipped too low
   D. Chin tipped too high

2. Identify the entity at arrows A.
   A. Torus palatinus
   B. Periapical cemental dysplasia

C. Complex odontoma

D. Soft tissue outline of the nose

3. What is the thick radiopaque band at arrows B?
   A. Chin rest, due to improper patient positioning
   B. Ghost image of the hyoid bone
   C. Orthodontic head gear
   D. Osteosclerosis or bone scar at a healed orthognathic surgical margin

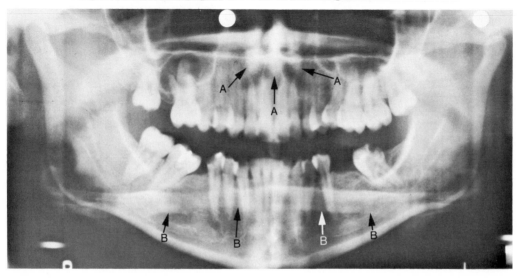

FIGURE 7–11

In looking at this radiograph, you will note that the patient has socket sclerosis in the mandibular molar area. The following question has two correct choices—try to pick them both. Which of the following conditions may be associated with socket sclerosis?
A. Renal disease
B. Intestinal malabsorption disorders
C. Liver disease
D. Endocrine problems

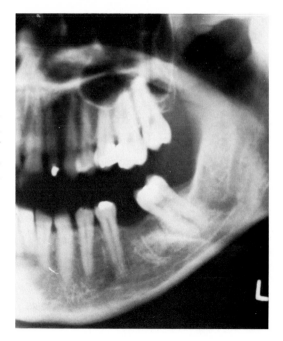

FIGURE 7–12

Look closely at these two radiographs of two different patients. In both cases the teeth are vital, and both patients are asymptomatic. The following is a list of four entities:
A. Incisive canal or incisive foramen
B. Incisive canal cyst (nasolacrimal duct cyst)
C. Lateral periodontal cyst
D. Primordial cyst of a mesiodens

For radiographs A and B, select one statement from the above that is most consistent with the radiograph. Only one statement is to be selected for each case, but the same statement may be selected both times.

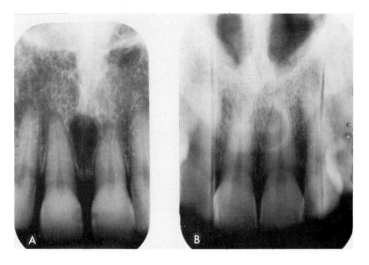

FIGURE 7–13

There are two questions pertaining to this radiograph.

1. What term best describes the position of the premolar at arrow A?
   A. Transposition
   B. Translocation
   C. Distal drift
   D. Migration

2. What is the cause of the radiolucent shadow obliterating all of the apices of the maxillary teeth?
   A. A large radiolucent lesion such as an odontogenic keratocyst
   B. Ghosts of the sinus air spaces
   C. Developer artifacts
   D. Palatoglossal air space due to tongue malpositioning

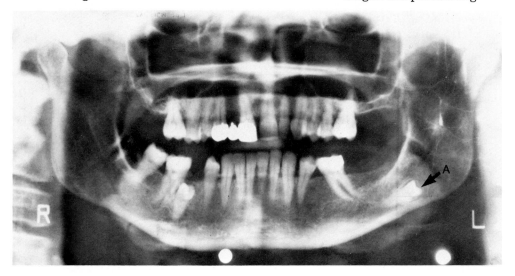

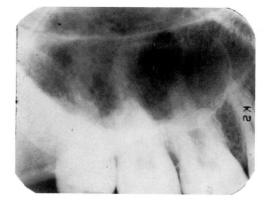

FIGURE 7–14

This periapical film was taken as part of a routine full mouth survey in an adult patient. All of the posterior teeth in this quadrant were free of caries and had never been restored. This patient had no other bony lesions and the urine was negative for Bence-Jones protein.

1. What is the most likely cause of the radiolucency at the apex of the first molar?
   A. Multiple or solitary myeloma
   B. Eosinophilic granuloma
   C. Sinus recess
   D. Lacrimal duct

2. What exposure error was made in taking this film?
   A. Excessive positive vertical angulation
   B. Excessive negative vertical angulation
   C. Improper horizontal angulation
   D. Placement of the film too high onto the palate

FIGURE 7–15

This patient is 22 years old and has lost most of his upper teeth owing to premature loosening and exfoliation. The patient has no caries, yet he has developed multiple periapical radiolucencies. Clinically the teeth look normal; however, the primary teeth had an opalescent appearance to them.

What is the patient's condition?
A. Amelogenesis imperfecta
B. Dentin dysplasia, type I
C. Dentin dysplasia, type II
D. Periapical cemental dysplasia, stage 1
E. Dentinogenesis imperfecta (hereditary opalescent dentin)

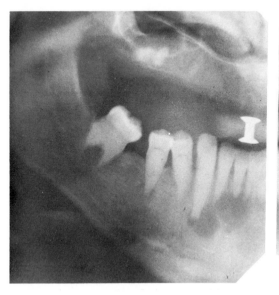
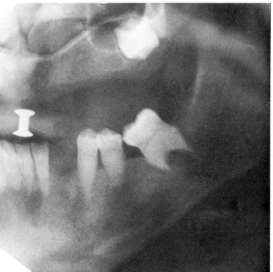

FIGURE 7–16

What is your impression of the radiopacity seen in the midline region?
A. Osteosclerosis
B. Condensing osteitis
C. Cementoma
D. Complex odontoma

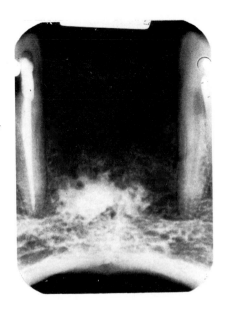

FIGURE 7-17

John Smith is a 45 year old white male who is currently asymptomatic. All four first bicuspids are missing, and all remaining teeth are vital.

1. What do you think the radiolucency at arrow A is?

   A. Incisive foramen

   B. Superior foramen of the incisive canal

   C. Incisive canal cyst (nasolacrimal duct cyst)

   D. Cementoma, stage 1 (osteolytic stage)

2. Look at the radiolucency at arrow A and, if possible, localize it to the labial side, the palatal side, or midway between the two.

   A. Labial

   B. In the middle

   C. Palatal

   D. Impossible to localize

3. Why do you suppose the roots of the lateral incisors are blunted and shortened?

   A. Previous orthodontic treatment

   B. Shovel-shaped incisor syndrome

   C. Idiopathic root resorption

   D. A previous lesion and its removal affected the teeth.

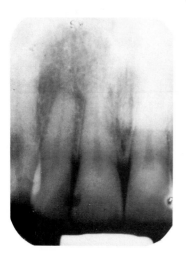
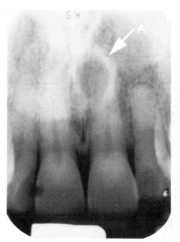
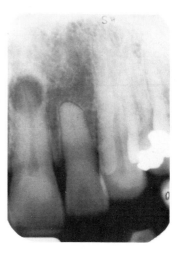

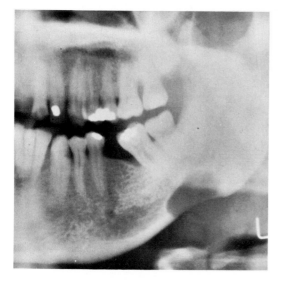

FIGURE 7-18

Here you can see a radiolucent lesion at the inferior border of the left side of the mandible. The patient, who is currently asymptomatic, is a 56 year old male. There was no history of trauma, and all the teeth are vital. What is the radiolucent lesion?

   A. Primordial cyst

   B. Metastatic disease

   C. Salivary gland depression

   D. Fibrous healing defect

FIGURE 7–19

This case involves a right-handed male patient of middle age. Upon interpreting this bitewing view, you note the distinct line extending across the cervical portion of the roots. The patient has no complaints of oral discomfort, nor was there any history of radiation therapy. What is the cause of this line at arrows A?

A. Chemical erosion
B. Toothbrush abrasion
C. Cervical caries
D. Horizontal root fractures

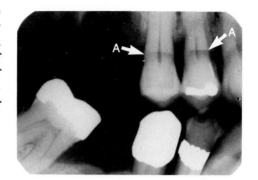

FIGURE 7–20

In this radiograph, the patient's midline is between the teeth labeled A and B. There is a normal complement of teeth, and mild crowding is present. Now look at tooth C. What term best describes the appearance of tooth C?

A. Concrescence
B. Gemination (schizodontism)
C. Fusion (synodontism)
D. Macrodontia

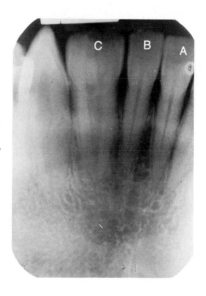

FIGURE 7–21

Look at this panoramic film. The problem is one of localization. As the consulting radiologist you are requested to determine whether the surgical approach for a ligation procedure on the maxillary left canine should be on the palatal or labial side.

Is the impacted left canine toward the palatal side, toward the labial side, in the middle, or impossible to localize?

A. Labial
B. Midway between the palatal and labial
C. Palatal
D. Impossible to localize

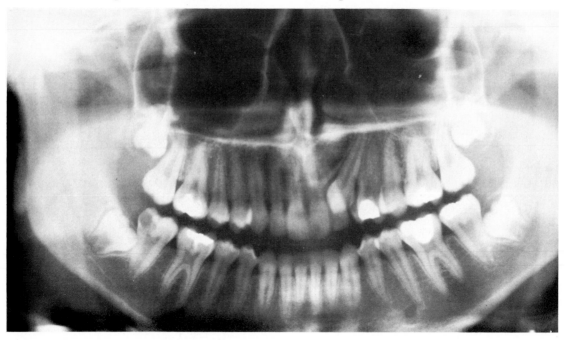

FIGURE 7–22

The patient is a 28 year old female. She was asymptomatic at the time of her examination; however, the panoramic radiograph showed a large lesion that was seen to be crossing the midline. There was no history of trauma. Biopsy of the lesion was carried out, and the biopsy results prompted an order for serum calcium studies. Serum calcium values were found to be normal. The lesion was excised, and the patient has not had a recurrence in the past 5 years.

1. From the list below, select three errors that occurred in the taking of this film.
   A. Chin too high
   B. Chin too low
   C. Palatoglossal airspace
   D. Partial denture left in
   E. Cotton roll or bite guide not used

2. From the history, what was the diagnosis?
   A. Central giant cell granuloma
   B. Hyperparathyroidism
   C. Traumatic cyst
   D. Odontogenic keratocyst

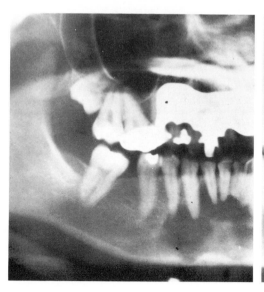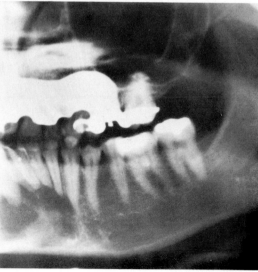

FIGURE 7–23

Endodontic work, which was completed some six years ago, is evident in these radiographs. The patient is currently asymptomatic. The tooth is not sensitive to percussion.

You will note that this figure has several labeled arrows pointing at specific entities. Match each label's letter (A, B, C, etc.) with the term that best describes what the letter's arrow (or group of arrows) is pointing at.

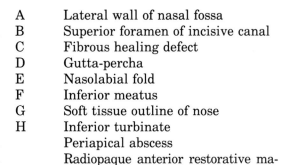

A	Lateral wall of nasal fossa
B	Superior foramen of incisive canal
C	Fibrous healing defect
D	Gutta-percha
E	Nasolabial fold
F	Inferior meatus
G	Soft tissue outline of nose
H	Inferior turbinate
	Periapical abscess
	Radiopaque anterior restorative material

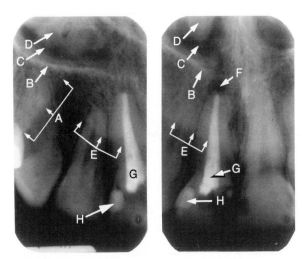

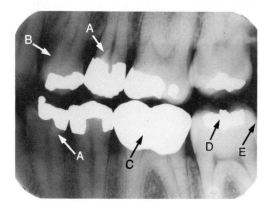

FIGURE 7–24

For this radiograph, match each of the letters in the left-hand column below with the term in the right-hand column that best describes what the letter's arrow is pointing at.

A	Enamel
B	Sclerotic dentin
C	Amalgam
D	Reparative dentin
E	Cast restoration
	Dentin
	Cervical burnout
	Caries

FIGURE 7–25

The patient, a Mexican-American female, is about 15 years old and her occlusion is normal. There was no history of crowding of the permanent teeth and she has never had any skeletal growth abnormality.

What is your diagnosis in this case? Remember—choose *the most* correct answer.

A. Orthodontic root resorption
B. Panoramic positioning error
C. Generalized microdontia
D. Shovel-shaped incisor syndrome

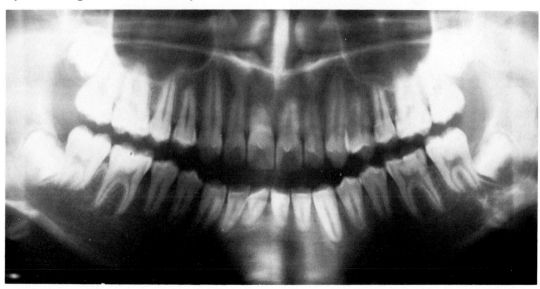

FIGURE 7–26

In this case, in which the patient was a 19 year old female, there were the following radiographic findings:

Generalized loss of the lamina dura
Ground glass pattern of alveolar bone
Severe erosion

The patient's serum calcium values tended to run in the high normal range, but she spilled calcium in her urine when she was placed on a low calcium diet.

1. Which of the following diagnostic possibilities would be suggested by the radiographic findings alone?

A. Fibrous dysplasia
B. Hyperparathyroidism
C. Paget disease
D. Dominant craniometaphyseal dysplasia
E. All of the above

2. Based upon the history, which of the specific diagnoses below would you select?

A. Fibrous dysplasia
B. Primary hyperparathyroidism
C. Secondary hyperparathyroidism (renal osteodystrophy)
D. Osteoporosis

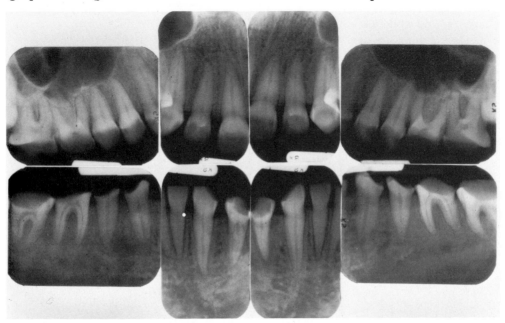

FIGURE 7–27

This is a radiograph of a resected specimen taken from a 37 year old white male. Based upon the radiograph, the following differential diagnosis was established:

Ameloblastoma
Odontogenic myxoma
Central giant cell granuloma
Central vascular lesion

Considering the history and treatment rendered, what do you think the diagnosis was?

A. Ameloblastoma
B. Odontogenic myxoma
C. Central giant cell granuloma
D. Aneurysmal bone cyst
E. Central vascular lesion

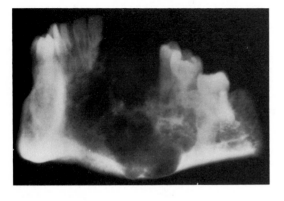

FIGURE 7–28

Note the radiopacity at the angle of the mandible. The patient was asymptomatic, had no systemic disorders or syndromes, and had no visible skin lesions. From the list below, select the two lesions that are the most probable causes of the radiopacity:

A. Osteoma
B. Sialolith
C. Phlebolith
D. Calcified lymph node
E. Cysticercosis

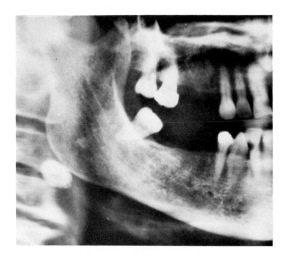

FIGURE 7–29

The film shows a radiolucent lesion and malpositioning of some teeth. The patient was an 18 year old female who was normal in every way except for a marked hypernasality in her speech.

1. What is the radiolucency in the left anterior maxilla?

    A. Fibrous healing defect (from orthognathic surgery)
    B. Globulomaxillary cyst
    C. Cleft palate
    D. Adenomatoid odontogenic tumor
    E. Incisive canal cyst

2. Note that the maxillary left first bicuspid and canine are not in their correct positions. What term best describes this finding?

    A. Ectopic eruption
    B. Distal drift
    C. Migration
    D. Transposition (translocation)

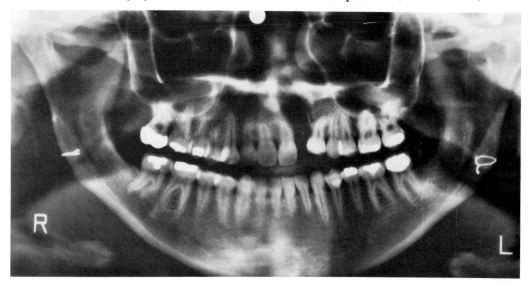

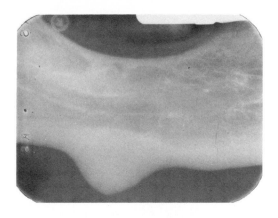

FIGURE 7-30

This case involves a 68 year old edentulous white male who had an easily palpable bump beneath the mandible. What term would *least* describe this lesion?

A. Exostosis
B. Osteoma
C. Mandibular torus
D. None of the above

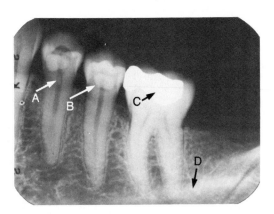

FIGURE 7-31

Each of this figure's lettered arrows points to a radiopaque entity. The letters appear below in the left column. Match each letter with the correct entity in the right column.

A	Pulp stone
B	Amalgam restoration
C	External oblique ridge
D	Cast gold restoration
	Tooth-colored filling material
	Internal oblique ridge

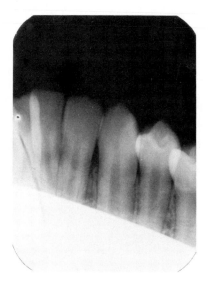

FIGURE 7-32

When this periapical film was taken, the long cone and lead apron were used as a precaution because the patient, a fully dentate 25 year old, was 2½ months pregnant. In your opinion, which *one* of the following errors occurred?

A. Rectangular cone cut
B. Partial denture left in
C. Film placed on top of tongue
D. Lead apron blocked beam

FIGURE 7-33

The patient is a 38 year old female who is currently asymptomatic. She has generalized moderate periodontal disease and she had a fair degree of calculus deposition about most of the teeth. Biopsy of the lesion revealed that it contained primarily fibrous connective tissue with some inflammatory elements.

What do you think this lesion represents?
A. Fibrous healing defect following surgical removal of the canine
B. Severe localized periodontitis due to local factors
C. Adult-onset periodontosis
D. Adenomatoid odontogenic tumor

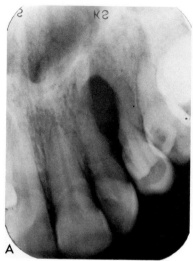
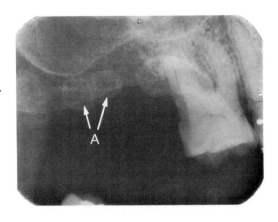

FIGURE 7-34

Which term best describes the two radiopacities at arrows A?
A. Antrolith(s)
B. Torus palatinus
C. Buccal exostoses
D. Phalangioma

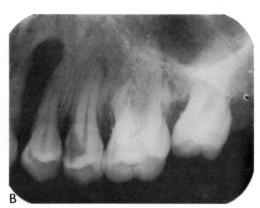

FIGURE 7–35

Well, here it is—the last one! And it's the one you've been waiting for.

The patient whose radiograph is shown here is an 18 year old white male. He has open fontanels, wormian bones, deficient clavicles, frontal bossing, and very few erupted permanent teeth. What's his condition?

A. Cleidocranial dysplasia
B. Gardner's syndrome
C. Cherubism
D. Idiopathic hyperdontia

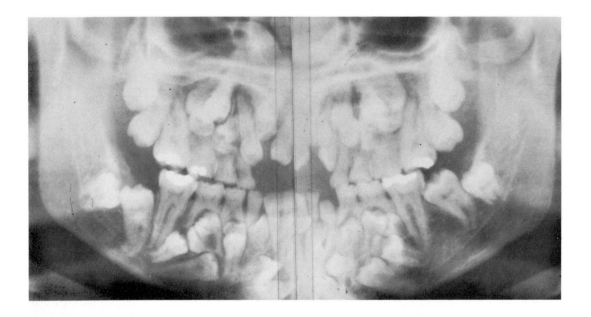

Answers

SECTION 1

FIGURE 1–1

1. Maxillary sinus
2. Nasal fossa
3. Superior foramen of the incisive canal
4. Incisive canal

FIGURE 1–2

1. Superior foramen of the incisive canal
2. Incisive canal

FIGURE 1–3

Inverted "Y." The floor of the nasal fossa and the maxillary sinus resemble the arms of the letter "Y," and the bony wall separating the two structures resembles the leg of that letter.

FIGURE 1–4

1. Sinus recess
2. A periapical granuloma, surgical defect, periapical cyst, or periapical abscess

FIGURE 1–5

The nasolabial fold

FIGURE 1–6

1. The nose
2. The median palatal suture
3. The incisive foramen

FIGURE 1–7

1. The tip of the nose
2. The peripheral outline of the nose

FIGURE 1–8

1. A nutrient canal
2. The maxillary sinus
3. The cortical plate of the anterior wall of the maxillary sinus
4. The maxillary antral mucosa

FIGURE 1–9

1. The zygomatic arch
2. The maxillary sinus (floor)
3. The coronoid process of the mandible

FIGURE 1–10

1. The lateral plate of the pterygoid process

2. The medial plate of the pterygoid process or the hamulus

FIGURE 1–11

1. Pterygoid complex
2. Temporal bone
3. Mandibular condyle
4. Zygomatic arch (zygomatic process of the temporal bone)

FIGURE 1–12

The nasolacrimal duct

FIGURE 1–13

1. The lateral fossa
2. A globulomaxillary cyst

FIGURE 1–14

1. The nasal fossa
2. Inferior turbinate
3. The nasal septum
4. The anterior nasal spine

FIGURE 1–15

1. The incisive foramen
2. The upper lip line

FIGURE 1–16

1. The nasal fossa
2. The maxillary sinus

FIGURE 1–17

1. Zygomatic process of the maxilla
2. Inferior border of the zygomatic arch (malar bone)
3. Maxillary tuberosity
4. The coronoid process of the mandible
5. The medial sigmoid depression

FIGURE 1–18

This is the incisive foramen (nasopalatine foramen). As it appears in this radiograph it could be incorrectly identified as an incisive canal cyst. Diagnosis should not be based on the radiograph alone.

FIGURE 1–19

The difference is in the angulation of the x-ray cone. In radiograph *A* the positive vertical angulation of the cone is less than that in radiograph *B*.

FIGURE 1–20

1. The zygomatic process of the maxilla
2. The soft-tissue shadow of the hamular notch

FIGURE 1–21

1. The external oblique ridge
2. The mandibular canal

FIGURE 1–22

The mental foramen. There has been a great deal of bone resorption, and the mental foramen now appears to be on the occlusal surface of the mandible.

FIGURE 1–23

You are correct if you said this is the mandibular anterior area. The next correct answer is that (1) is the shadow of the lower lip. The round radiopaque area is the genial tubercle, with the lingual foramen showing as a small radiolucency at its center.

FIGURE 1–24

1. The mental foramen
2. The submandibular fossa

FIGURE 1–25

Nutrient canals

FIGURE 1–26

1. The inferior cortex of the mandible
2. The submandibular fossa
3. The mandibular (inferior alveolar) canal
4. The internal oblique ridge (mylohyoid line)

FIGURE 1–27

1. The external oblique ridge
2. The internal oblique ridge (mylohyoid line)
3. The mandibular (inferior alveolar) canal

FIGURE 1–28

1. The lower lip line
2. The mental ridge

3. The lingual canal
4. The cortical plate of the lower border of the mandible

FIGURE 1–29

The arrows are pointing at the anterior border of the tongue. The film was positioned over the tongue.

FIGURE 1–30

1. Lateral wall of the nasal fossa
2. Medial wall of the maxillary sinus
3. Inverted "Y"
4. Superior foramen of the incisive canal
5. Nasal septum
6. Nasal fossa

This is a maxillary anterior occlusal view.

FIGURE 1–31

1. Mental ridge
2. Canal of the lingual artery and vein
3. Inferior cortex of the mandible
4. Internal oblique ridge (mylohyoid line)
5. External oblique ridge
6. Soft tissue of the lower lip
7. Soft tissue of the tongue

This is a mandibular anterior occlusal view.

FIGURE 1–32

1. Mandibular condyle
2. Mandibular fossa (glenoid fossa)
3. Articular eminence
4. Zygomatic arch (malar bone)
5. Pterygomaxillary fissure
6. Posterior wall of the maxillary sinus
7. Zygomatic process of the maxilla
8. Ghost image of the contralateral hard palate
9. Actual hard palate
10. Floor of the maxillary sinus
11. Anterior wall of the maxillary sinus (lateral wall of the nasal fossa)
12. Nasal septum
13. Nasal fossa
14. Maxillary sinus
15. Orbit
16. Panoramic innominate line
17. Coronoid process of the mandible
18. Sigmoid notch
19. Posterior border of the ramus

20. Gonial angle
21. Anterior border of the pancentric patient positioning bar
22. Ghost image of the "R" marker
23. Body of the hyoid bone
24. Mental foramen
25. Mandibular (inferior alveolar) canal
26. Ghost image of the "L" marker
27. Soft tissue of the ear lobe
28. Soft palate
29. Maxillary tuberosity
30. External oblique ridge

FIGURE 1–33

1. External auditory canal
2. Mandibular condyle
3. Variation of normal representing a depression in the head of the condyle
4. Articular eminence
5. Zygomatic arch (malar bone)
6. Lateral pterygoid plate
7. Posterior wall of the maxillary sinus
8. Panoramic innominate line
9. Orbit
10. Inferior border of the orbit
11. Inferior border of the maxillary sinus
12. Maxillary sinus
13. Actual image of the right side of the hard palate
14. Ghost image of the left side of the palate
15. Middle meatus
16. Common meatus
17. Soft tissue of tip of the nose
18. Pterygomaxillary fissure
19. Coronoid process of the mandible
20. Sigmoid notch
21. Posterior border of the ramus
22. Gonial angle
23. Actual image of the "L" marker
24. Double image of the body of the hyoid bone
25. External oblique ridge
26. Mandibular (inferior alveolar) canal
27. Ear lobe
28. Anterior tubercle of C-1
29. Medial sigmoid depression
30. Soft tissue outline of the lips

FIGURE 1–34

1. Frontal sinus
2. Outer table
3. Inner table
4. Coronal suture
5. Lambdoid suture
6. Occipital area
7. Mastoid air cells
8. Petrous ridge
9. Calcified petroclinoid ligament
10. Dorsum sellae
11. Posterior clinoid process
12. Pituitary fossa
13. Anterior clinoid process
14. Sphenoid sinus
15. Ethmoid air cells
16. Cerebral surfaces of the orbital plates
17. Anterior nasal spine
18. Zygomatic process of the maxilla
19. Maxillary sinus
20. Hard palate (floor of the sinus)
21. Pterygomaxillary fissure
22. Air space of the oropharynx
23. Dorsal surface of the tongue
24. Anterior tubercle of the atlas (C-1)
25. Odontoid process of the axis (C-2)
26. Atlas (C-1)
27. Posterior pharyngeal wall
28. Axis (C-2)
29. Body of the third cervical vertebra
30. Gonial angle of the left mandible

FIGURE 1–35

1. Mastoid air cells
2. Petrous ridge
3. Lateral border of the orbit
4. Supraorbital ridge
5. Frontal sinus
6. Outer table
7. Inner table
8. Ethmoid air cells
9. Nasal septum
10. Inferior turbinate
11. Common meatus
12. Inferior meatus
13. Anterior nasal spine
14. Joint between C-1 and C-2
15. Lateral mass of C-1
16. Floor of the nasal fossa
17. Zygomatic arch (malar bone)
18. Odontoid process of C-2
19. Body of the mandible
20. Ramus of the mandible
21. Sphenoid sinus

FIGURE 1–36

1. Maxillary sinus
2. Coronoid process of the mandible
3. Zygomatic arch
4. Lateral border of the orbit
5. Orbit
6. Supraorbital ridge
7. Frontal sinus
8. Ethmoid air cells
9. Nasal septum
10. Sphenoid sinus
11. Odontoid process of C-2
12. Body of the mandible
13. Gonial angle
14. Posterior border of the ramus
15. Mastoid air cells
16. Joint between C-1 and C-2
17. Infraorbital foramen

FIGURE 1–37

1. Mastoid air cells
2. External auditory meatus
3. Jugular foramen
4. Internal auditory canal

5. Head of the mandibular condyle
6. Foramen spinosum
7. Foramen ovale
8. Angle of the mandible
9. Medial aspect of mandibular ramus
10. Posterior border of hard palate
11. Coronoid process of mandible
12. Anterior ethmoid air cells
13. Vomer and perpendicular plate of ethmoid
14. Lateral wall of nasal fossa (medial wall of maxillary sinus)
15. Lateral wall of maxillary sinus
16. Zygomatic process of maxilla
17. Zygomatic arch (malar bone)
18. Posterior ethmoid air cells
19. Foramen magnum
20. Odontoid process of C-2
21. Sphenoid sinus
22. Maxillary sinus
23. Nasal fossa

Structure #17, the malar bone, will show only if lower exposures are used, including a decrease in kVp and mAs.

SECTION 2

FIGURE 2–1

Adumbration (cervical burn-out). This usually occurs when the horizontal angle of the beam is not directed through the contact areas of the teeth being radiographed. This "off angle" may be in a mesial or distal direction and causes the buccal and lingual segments of the cervical portion of the teeth to appear to be separated. This produces a relative radiolucency that may be mistaken for cervical or root caries. Adumbration may be identified by the radiographic appearance or by repeating the radiograph using the proper horizontal angulation. Clinical inspection is helpful in ruling out caries.

FIGURE 2–2

Phalangioma (patient's finger)

FIGURE 2–3

1. **Cone cut**

2. The spot on the left-hand side is a clip mark from the processing rack; the spot on the edentulous ridge is an amalgam fragment (amalgam tattoo).

FIGURE 2–4

While the film was in the developing solution **another film stuck to it.** Owing to surface tension between the two films, only one side of the film double emulsion was processed in this area; thus, a lighter image was produced.

FIGURE 2–5

This indicates an **improper horizontal angulation** of the radiographic beam in relation to these teeth.

FIGURE 2–6

1. Failure to place the film sufficiently apically

2. Inadequate **vertical** angulation of the radiographic beam

FIGURE 2–7

By failure to expose the film. This occurs when the time-exposure button is not depressed long enough to make an adequate exposure.

The film can also turn out this way if it is accidentally placed in the fixer solution first. The image is then completely wiped off the film.

FIGURE 2–8

1. **Patient movement**
2. **Film movement**
3. **X-ray machine movement**

FIGURE 2–9

1. **Grainy**
2. This will occur if the developer solution is too warm. The optimal temperature is 68° F when manual processing solutions are used.

FIGURE 2–10

Developer

FIGURE 2–11

Excessive curving of the posterior half of the film, which is usually due to excessive digital pressure by the patient as he is holding the film.

FIGURE 2–12

1. **Foreshortening** of the roots and superimposition of the zygomatic arch over the maxillary molar apices
2. **Excessive positive vertical angulation**

FIGURE 2–13

Handling of the film with **fluoride-contaminated fingers.** Contamination from developer solution will give the same results.

FIGURE 2–14

Fixer

FIGURE 2–15

Congratulations—you're right if you said **foreshortening.**

FIGURE 2–16

This is due to **dimensional distortion,** which is an inherent error when the bisecting angle radiographic technique is used.

FIGURE 2–17

Elongation. This error was made either by using inadequate positive vertical angulation of the radiographic beam; or by failing to have the ala-tragus plane or occlusal plane parallel to the floor in the bisecting angle technique and then not using sufficient positive vertical angulation of the radiographic beam.

FIGURE 2–18

1. **Elongation**
2. **Fingernail artifact**
Hurrah! You did it!
Note that this same artifact will occur as a result of crimping of the film as the film is handled or removed from the packet before processing.

FIGURE 2–19

The error is **magnification,** which is rather rare. It is usually seen when the film-to-object distance is increased and a divergent beam such as exists in some short or pointed cones is used. It also occurs as a result of machine movement during exposure of the film. Machine movement causes an effective increase in the target size, thus producing a magnified image with a fuzzy outline, which is due to the increased penumbra that also occurs.

FIGURE 2–20

1. **Insufficient exposure time**
2. **Insufficient milliamperage setting (mAs)**
3. **Insufficient mAs factor** relative to the patient's bone density
4. **Inadequate development**
5. **Weak or depleted developer solution**
6. **Insufficient kilovoltage**
7. **Expired or aged film**

FIGURE 2–21

1. **Zygomatic arch**

2. Through excessive positive vertical angulation of the radiographic beam

FIGURE 2–22

A double exposure

FIGURE 2–23

The rubber roller of the automatic processor. The rubber can actually come off the rollers and adhere to the processed radiograph.

If you look closely, you can also see static electricity superimposed over the mesial root of the mandibular molar.

FIGURE 2–24

This line is radiopaque. Bending the film clinically produces a radiolucent line (see the top left corner of Fig. 2–18). **This artifact is produced in automatic processing machines.** The cause of this occurrence is not well understood, but the artifact probably results from use of the bent edge of a film as the leading edge in the automatic processor. The ragged edge in the lower right-hand corner represents torn emulsion.

FIGURE 2–25

1. It was **overexposed** to radiation.
2. It was **overdeveloped.**
3. The **developer solution** was improperly mixed, so that an over-concentrated solution was inadvertently produced.
4. There was **a light leak** in the film-processing darkroom.

FIGURE 2–26

Overlapping of the contacts. This error was made by **improper horizontal angulation** of the beam.

FIGURE 2–27

Scratching of the emulsion

Note the film fogging, which may be produced by a darkroom light leak, a safelight that is too close to the counter-top, an improper filter on the safelight, a scattering of secondary radiation, chemicals, or the aging of the film (outdated film).

FIGURE 2–28

The film was reversed when placed in the patient's mouth. The tab side of the film packet was facing the beam. The x-rays were partially absorbed by the lead backing; thus the characteristic "tire tracks" or "herring bone" pattern was produced on the film. The film therefore appears light, underexposed, and foggy.

FIGURE 2–29

The lower edge of the film was not placed parallel to the occlusal surfaces of the teeth. Actually, as often happens, the film was properly placed but was moved by the patient just prior to exposure.

FIGURE 2–30

Inadequate fixation. The film was not left in the fixer long enough after development.

FIGURE 2–31

1. Use of **outdated film**
2. **Storage** of the film in a warm place
3. Exposure of the film to **scatter radiation**
4. **Light leaks** in the darkroom
5. Excessive proximity of the **safelight** to the film
6. **Improper filtration** on the safelight for the type of film used
7. Use of **too strong a bulb** for the safelight filter used

You knew these, didn't you? Say "Yes." You'll make us feel better.

FIGURE 2–32

1. **A metal or leaded glass fragment** imbedded in soft tissue overlying the lesion
2. **A metallic object inside a pointed cone**
3. **Scratched emulsion**
4. **A metal fragment imbedded in the bone,** which is the cause of the lesion
5. **A fixer artifact**

In fact, this radiopacity represents scratched emulsion over the superior foramen of the incisive canal. What do you think of that?

FIGURE 2–33

A—**Fixer artifact**

B—**Ethiodized oil** used for opacification of salivary gland ducts and some radiolucent lesions

C—**Shotgun pellet**

Other possible causes:

a. **Air bubble.** With improper agitation the bubble adheres to the surface of the film. This portion of the film is not developed properly.

b. **Soft-tissue calcifications**

FIGURE 2–34

These are **streaks of developer** from a clip that was previously used in concentrated solutions. Be sure to wash the film-holding clips thoroughly in clean water before reusing them.

FIGURE 2–35

The patient's name was written on the front of the packet with an ordinary **ball point pen** prior to exposure.

FIGURE 2–36

1. **Zygomatic arch**
2. **Excessive positive vertical angulation of the x-ray cone**

FIGURE 2–37

Reticulation. This is a cracking of the film emulsion due to extreme differences in processing-solution temperatures. The tap water temperature was much cooler than the developer and fixer solution temperatures.

FIGURE 2–38

1. **Failure to stir the developer solution.** The solution was weaker at the top than further down.
2. **Insufficient solution in the fixer tank.** The upper portion of the film was not fixed, thus producing the dark line.

FIGURE 2–39

This film was placed in a manner similar to that for an occlusal film and was taken at a high angle, so that it resembles a periapical view. When biting on the film pack the patient used excessive force, so that at the points of contact of the teeth the film emulsion was crimped. The radiolucent "lesion-like" artifacts appeared after development.

FIGURE 2–40

Developer splashed on the film prior to developing.

FIGURE 2–41

1. **Static electricity**
2. **Fingernail artifact**
3. Film crimping artifact

FIGURE 2–42

Rectangular cone cut

FIGURE 2–43

If you said **developer artifact,** you are absolutely right!

FIGURE 2–44

Well, if you chose **fixer artifact,** you are not only right, but now you know you also learned the material very well!

FIGURE 2–45

Denture with porcelain teeth left in

FIGURE 2-46

1. **Patient too far forward** in the machine

2. a. **Narrow anterior teeth**
   b. **Superimposition of the cervical spine** on the ramus

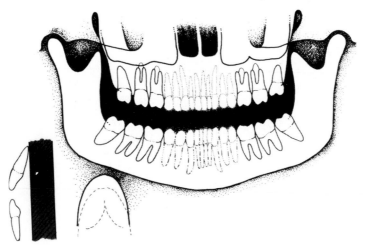

FIGURE 2-47

1. **Patient too far back in the machine**
2. a. **Wide anterior teeth**

b. **Loss of the apical image** of the maxillary or mandibular teeth

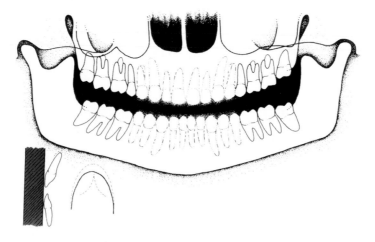

FIGURE 2–48

1. The patient's **head was twisted.**
2. a. **Narrow teeth on one side** of the image and **wider teeth on the other side of the image**

   b. A **narrow ramus on one side** of the image and a **wider ramus on the other side** of the image

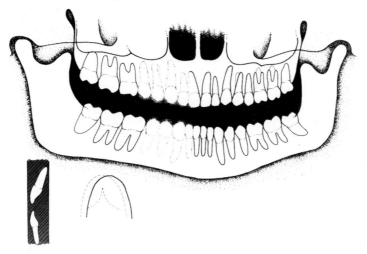

FIGURE 2–49

1. The patient's **chin was tipped too low.**
2. a. **Excessive smile line** when looking at the teeth

   b. **Loss of the apical image** at the mandibular incisors

   c. **Loss of the TMJ's off the top** of the image

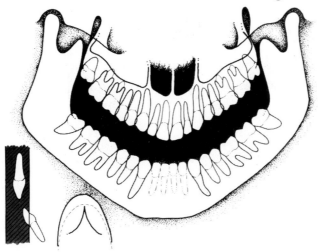

FIGURE 2–50

1. The patient's **chin was tipped too high.**
   2. a. **Reverse smile line** or flat occlusal plane

b. **Loss of the apical image at the maxillary incisors**
c. **Superimposition of the hard palate shadow** on the maxillary apices
d. **Tendency to lose the TMJ's off the edges of the image**

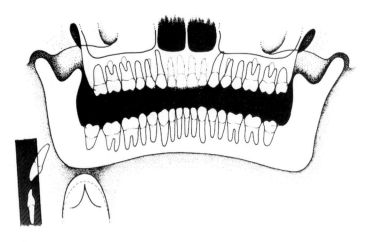

FIGURE 2–51

1. The patient **bent the neck while slumping** in the machine.

2. **Superimposition of the ghost image of the spine** in the anterior midline of the image

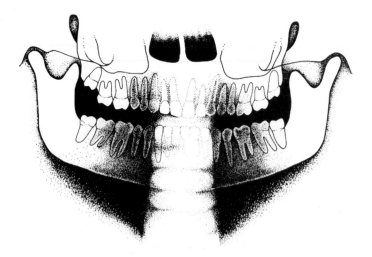

FIGURE 2–52

1. **Napkin chain** or **neck chain** error
2. **Superimposition of an inverted V-shaped ghost image of the chain** in the anterior mandibular area

FIGURE 2–53

1. **Film exposed to light** before processing
2. "Image" nil on light-exposed portion of film. Remember: **lock the darkroom door;** keep work involving regular lights separated from darkroom work.

FIGURE 2–54

1. **Protective apron shoulder strap artifact**
2. **A ghost image of each of the shoulder straps** in the right and left mandibular bicuspid regions
   Note: In sit-down machines, the shoulder straps tend to ride up onto the neck into the path of the beam when the patient sits down on the apron.

FIGURE 2–55

1. **Tongue air-space error**
2. **A black horizontal band obliterates the periapical region of the maxillary teeth.**

Note: The patient should be asked to hold the tongue tight up against the palate as occurs in swallowing.

FIGURE 2–56

1. **Not starting at home base**
2. **A portion of the film is blank, and a portion of the image of the jaws is missing.**
   Note: Some machines can be activated even when the cassette has not been been rotated to the correct starting point.

FIGURE 2–57

1. a. **Cassette hung up.**
   b. **Patient moved.**
2. a. When the cassette hangs up, usually in an item of clothing, the machine stops its rotation movement but continues to expose, thus producing the **dark vertical band representing an overexposed area.**
   b. **With subsequent patient movement, the remainder of the structures are in an incorrect relationship.**

Note: Cassette hang-ups and patient movement represent failure of the operator to check clothing or to adequately explain the function of the machine to the patient.

SECTION 3

FIGURE 3–1

1. a. **Amalgam**
   b. **Gold foil**
2. a. **Silicate**
   b. **Silicophosphate cement**
   c. **Acrylic**
   d. **Composite resin**

FIGURE 3–2

1. a. **Chrome cobalt (or other alloy)**
   b. **Gold**
2. **Acrylic**
3. **Radiopaque cement**

FIGURE 3–3

Porcelain jacket crown

FIGURE 3–4

1. **Amalgam at the apex**
2. **Gutta-percha**
3. **Cast gold post and core**
4. **Porcelain jacket or porcelain fused to gold full crown**

FIGURE 3–5

Acrylic

FIGURE 3–6

1. **Porcelain**
2. **Platinum foil** (used to plate the die during construction of the porcelain jacket crown)
   3. a. **Gutta-percha** (left central incisor)
      b. **Silver alloy** pit restoration (left central incisor)
   4. **Bending** of the corners of the film

FIGURE 3–7

1. **Leaded glass fragment embedded in lower lip**
   2. a. **Scratched emulsion**
      b. **Metallic object** trapped inside the pointed cone
      c. **Amalgam tattoo**
      d. **Metal fragment** such as a bullet fragment or bird shot

FIGURE 3–8

1. **He is 6½ to 8 years old.** The child must be more than 5½ because the centrals have erupted; he must be less than 11½ years old because the cuspids have not yet erupted. He must be more than 6, because the laterals have begun to erupt, but less than 9, because the laterals have not yet fully erupted nor is root formation complete.
2. **Lingual version,** which is apparent from the fact that the bite plane seen on this film is used to correct this condition

FIGURE 3–9

1. **Stainless steel wire splint**
2. This appears to be a **young** patient because relatively large pulp canals and relatively good periodontal support are evident.
3. **Trauma** to the anterior teeth resulted in loosening of the teeth, requiring temporary stabilization.

FIGURE 3–10

1. **An ivory rubber dam frame**
2. **An endodontic file**
3. **An ivory #9 endodontic clamp**
4. **Silver alloy restorations**
5. **The tip of the mosquito forceps that were used as a film holder**

FIGURE 3–11

1. a. Lateral incisor—**retrograde silver alloy**
   b. Cuspid—**gutta-percha technique**
2. It had an obliterated pulp canal and a porcelain jacket crown.

FIGURE 3–12

Open-faced stainless steel crowns

FIGURES 3–13 THROUGH 3–37

Remember, answers are from left to right.

Figure 3–13—**pin-type** implant and a **porcelain fused to gold fixed bridge**

Figure 3–14—**a blade implant** and an **amalgam fragment**

Figure 3–15—a **cotton roll, rubber,** and a **metallic bite-block**

Figure 3–16—a **bite-wing tab**

Figure 3–17—a **retentive pin** and a **broken burr tip,** now perforating the tooth, that was used to prepare a pin hole

Figure 3–18—a **porcelain tooth, wire mesh** to strengthen the palate of the denture, and a **metallic pin** for the anterior porcelain denture tooth

Figure 3–19—a **wrought wire clasp** for an acrylic partial denture

Figure 3–20—the **maxillary sinus septum** (not to be confused with endodontic materials)

Figure 3–21—**gutta-percha,** a **broken file or lentula,** and **gold casting**

Figure 3–22—**silver points** and a **gutta-percha point**

Figure 3–23—the tip of **college pliers** used as a film holder (cotton pliers)

Figure 3–24—**amalgam, gold casting, and porcelain facing**

Figure 3–25—an **alloy** partial denture framework that has acrylic prosthetic teeth that are not visible

Figure 3–26—an **alloy** partial denture framework, **porcelain teeth**, and gold casting

Figure 3–27—**eyeglasses** (glass lenses) and the **metallic frames** for the lenses

Figure 3–28—**Porcelain denture teeth**

Figure 3–29—**Wire** (for fracture reduction)

Figure 3–30—an **orthodontic bracket, wire** (for tooth separation), and an **orthodontic band**

Figure 3–31—**gold casting, acrylic facing** (not visible), and **calculus** (note the calculus adhering to the gingival area of the acrylic facing)

Figure 3–32—a **cement base, gold casting,** and **composite resin**

Figure 3–33—older, **radiolucent tooth-colored filling material** and **newer, radiopaque material**

Figure 3–34—**cast gold alloy,** a **cement base,** and **amalgam**

Figure 3–35—**gauze,** a **suture needle,** and the **tip of mosquito forceps**

Figure 3–36—**porcelain,** the **metal alloy** palate of a partial denture, **cement,** and an **acrylic crown** (not visible)

Figure 3–37—a **vitreous carbon implant** (not visible) with a **gold alloy post** and an acrylic temporary crown (not visible)

FIGURE 3–38

1. Zinc oxide–eugenol **cement** and formocresol
2. A **stainless steel crown**

FIGURE 3–39

A **calcium hydroxide** pulp cap and a temporary **cement** seal

FIGURE 3–40

The patient suffered from emphysema. He carried with him a portable oxygen tank with its tubing attached. You see the **image of the plastic tubing.**

SECTION 4

FIGURE 4–1

1. **Dens in dente**
2. **Obliteration** of the root canal space

FIGURE 4–2

1. Mandibular first permanent molar restored with **amalgam** and a **cement base**
2. There is evidence of **secondary dentin** formation beneath the mesial pulpal floor. The tooth is **"submerged"** with respect to the adjacent teeth. There is evidence of external **resorption** of the roots in the bifurcation area with bone replacement. In these areas, there are no discernible periodontal membrane spaces, so that the tooth is partially **ankylosed.** There is evidence of **osteosclerosis** or **focal sclerosing osteomyelitis** of undetermined origin.

FIGURE 4–3

1. **Hereditary hypohidrotic ectodermal dysplasia**
2. **Incontinentia pigmenti** and **chondroectodermal dysplasia**

FIGURE 4–4

1. **Autogenous transplant** of the developing third molar to replace the first molar
2. Notice the **flat mesial surfaces** of both the second molar and the transplanted third molar. This flattening was done in order to accommodate the transplanted tooth. Note **decalcification** on the mesial of the second molar and on the distal of the transplanted tooth. On the mesial and occlusal surfaces of the transplanted tooth **caries** is evident. There is an **open contact** and resultant early signs of **destruction of the interseptal cortical bone.** As is common with transplanted and reimplanted teeth, there is almost complete **resorption of the roots,** and in some areas the remaining tooth structure appears to be continuous with the surrounding bone, thus indicating **ankylosis.** The **pulp chamber** appears to be completely **obliterated.**

FIGURE 4–5

1. **Cleidocranial dysplasia**
2. There is a relative **lack of cellular**

cementum on the roots, a deficiency that may in some way be connected with the delayed eruption.

FIGURE 4–6

1. **Congenitally missing** permanent mandibular central incisors
2. **Rieger's syndrome**
3. Affected children appear normal in every other way; however, **cataracts** develop insidiously by the age of 6 to 8 due to **congenital glaucoma.** An important sign of glaucoma in these children is an excessive discomfort in reaction to the operatory light if it is inadvertently directed in their eyes (photophobia).

FIGURE 4–7

1. **Enamel pearl** (enameloma)
2. **Ankylosis**
3. **Osteosclerosis** (bone scar) or **focal sclerosing osteomyelitis** (condensing osteitis)
Note: The first occurs in the absence of infection, whereas the last is a proliferative response to a low-grade infection, often of pulpal origin.

FIGURE 4–8

1. **"Submerged" tooth.** This is due to the difference in height between the deciduous and permanent occlusal planes and also to the retention and ankylosis of the deciduous second molar associated with the congenitally missing permanent second bicuspid.
2. **Deep occlusal caries**

FIGURE 4–9

Toothbrush abrasion. The characteristic features are the sharp, thin, radiolucent line crossing the mesial-to-distal width of the tooth in the cervical area and a distinct V-shaped defect seen in the cervical third of the crown. This latter characteristic can be visualized only when the tooth, film, and beam are exactly aligned.

FIGURE 4–10

1. a. **Attrition**
   b. **Pulp calcification** in the first and second bicuspids

c. **Calculus** in the first and second bicuspids. (Note the unusual linear pattern.)
d. **Supernumerary roots** in the first and second bicuspids
2. **Generally indistinct lamina dura** and **horizontal bone loss**
3. **Bending of the film.** In order to accommodate the film in the patient's mouth, the lower mesial corner was bent, thus producing a "fuzzed-out" appearance of the bone in this area.

FIGURE 4–11

Tapered
Easy so far? Go on, there's more.

FIGURE 4–12

1. **Taurodontism**
2. a. **Tricho-dento-osseous syndrome**
   b. **Felty's syndrome**

FIGURE 4–13

1. **Supernumerary mandibular bicuspid tooth**
2. **Gardner's syndrome** and **cleidocranial dysplasia**
Note: The finding of supernumerary teeth does not necessarily imply that a concurrent syndrome or condition exists.

FIGURE 4–14

1. **Osteogenesis imperfecta**
2. **Dentinogenesis imperfecta** (dentinal dysplasia, type I)
3. **Early obliteration of the pulp and root canals** and **relatively less enamel** due to flaking caused by a defective dentinoenamel junction. Additional features, not seen here, are bulbous crowns with narrow shortened roots and root fractures.

FIGURE 4–15

A paramolar

FIGURE 4–16

1. **Radiation therapy**
2. a. **Radiation stunting.** The large dosages of radiation required during treatment caused injury to the developing teeth.

b. **Delayed eruption.** Although radiation often has this effect, the teeth usually do eventually erupt.

FIGURE 4–17

Supernumerary lateral incisor

FIGURE 4–18

1. In the mandibular second bicuspid there is **internal resorption** possibly due to a reactive hyperplastic pulp producing an odontoclastic response. Note the secondary dentin under the distal portion of the restoration and possible periapical involvement. In the mandibular first molar there is complete **obliteration of the coronal portion of the pulp** due to a reactive pulp producing an odontoblastic response. Note the defective distal margin of the restoration.

2. **One should treat both teeth with endodontic therapy.** The bicuspid should be treated in order to remove the hyperplastic pulp before a perforation occurs. The molar should be treated in order to remove the pulp before mechanical access to the canals and mechanical manipulation of the canals becomes impossible. The latter mode of therapy in this situation remains controversial.

FIGURE 4–19

1. In the **mandibular molar region**
2. **An unerupted molar**
3. a. **External resorption** of the occlusal area
   b. **Complete pulpal obliteration**
   c. **Ankylosis**
4. By **observation.** Removal would be difficult, and there does not appear to be any significant active pathologic process associated with the tooth or surrounding bone.

FIGURE 4–20

1. a. The **foramen of the nutrient canal**
   b. The **mental foramen**
2. Rapid **orthodontic** tooth movement. Notice that one of the bicuspids has been extracted. The net result is external root resorption resulting in shortened, blunted roots.

3. Obliteration of the pulp chamber in the bicuspid. Note the absence of caries.

FIGURE 4–21

1. **Dentin dysplasia, type I**
2. a. **Normal-sized crowns** with **normal enamel and dentin**
   b. Very **short blunted or pointed molar roots**
   c. **Tapered bicuspid and incisor roots**
   d. **Pulp obliteration**
   e. **Pulp stones**
   f. **Horizontal radiolucent lines**
   g. **Idiopathic periapical radiolucencies**
   h. **Early loosening and exfoliation of the permanent teeth**
3. **Normal**

FIGURE 4–22

1. A **supernumerary root** on the mandibular first bicuspid
2. **Nutrient canal**

FIGURE 4–23

1. A **rotated** right central incisor
2. **Pulp stones** in the right central and lateral incisors
3. **Horizontal bone loss** about the right central and lateral incisors
4. **Hypercementosis** of the mandibular right cuspid

FIGURE 4–24

This is a **horizontally impacted and possibly migrated tooth.** There is evidence of external resorption, especially of the coronal and apical portions of this tooth. These areas appear to be **ankylosed.** The tooth is located in the **mandibular midline area.**

FIGURE 4–25

1. **Mesiodens** (supernumerary central incisor)
2. **Palatally.** The closer an object is to the film the more radiopaque it will be. Compare the enamel of this tooth to the enamel of the central incisors.
3. a. By taking a radiograph using the maxillary crossfire occlusal view

b. By varying the vertical angulation (see Section 6, Buccal Object Rule)

c. By varying the horizontal angulation (see Section 6, Buccal Object Rule)

FIGURE 4–26

Transposition (translocation). Notice that the permanent lateral incisor is missing and the deciduous lateral incisor has been exfoliated. The permanent first bicuspid is erupting into the position of the permanent lateral incisor.

FIGURE 4–27

1. **Talon cusp**
2. **"Double" dens in dente**
3. **Prophylactic restoration** of the mesial and distal pits.

FIGURE 4–28

1. The **lateral canal**
2. **Mandibular lingual tori**

FIGURE 4–29

Bilateral impacted bicuspids or supernumerary bicuspids or both. Notice that the crowns are well demarcated by a radiolucent line that represents the follicular sac of the teeth.

FIGURE 4–30

Mamelons. Remember these from dental anatomy?

FIGURE 4–31

1. A **double-rooted lower cuspid**
2. a. **Abrupt diminution of the root canal space**
   b. **Several smaller root canal spaces**
   c. **Double periodontal membrane space** that mimics root fracture. Given these findings, one must realize that several other teeth in this radiograph may have supernumerary roots or bifurcation of the root canal space within the same root. These possibilities are important when endodontic therapy is being considered.

FIGURE 4–32

1. a. **External resorption** is present.
   b. There is a **residual periapical pathologic condition** or a **fibrous healing defect** if a resection was performed.
2. a. **Porcelain jacket crown**
   b. Prefabricated **screw-type** core

FIGURE 4–33

1. **Eight years** old, plus or minus one year
2. **Enamel hypoplasia,** environmental type. The subtypes are classified according to etiology, the most likely etiology here being exanthematous fevers or a nutritional deficiency during the first year of life. In some cases the actual cause may never be determined, whereas in other cases cause is determined with the help of a history and previous radiographs.
3. The **permanent lateral incisor, the cuspid, and the six-year molar.** The first bicuspid may be involved.

FIGURE 4–34

1. **Toothbrush abrasion**
2. **Foreshortening** due to using too steep or positive a vertical angle or not having the ala-tragus plane of the patient's head parallel to the floor when the film was exposed.

We knew you would get these two answers—you've seen them before!

FIGURE 4–35

1. **Bulimia**
2. The patient will "binge," sometimes consuming up to 10,000 calories in one session, and then voluntarily "purge" all of the food eaten. Some patients resort to laxative abuse as a means of purging; most simply throw up, subjecting the teeth to the passage of vomitus, and **it is the acid from the stomach contents that damages the teeth.**
3. **Chemical erosion**
4. **Perimyolysis.** Note the "sculptured" appearance of the cervical region.

Note: Affected patients eventually have restorative failures. Great benefit can be obtained by immediate rinsing with antacids.

FIGURE 4–36

Diastema. In this region distal to the cuspid in the mandible, this is known as the primate space in the primary dentition only.

FIGURE 4–37

Dilaceration. Note the "double" PDM space.

FIGURE 4–38

It is the **developing third molar.**

FIGURE 4–39

Distal drift

FIGURE 4–40

1. During the **first year of life**
2. **Enamel hypoplasia** of the maxillary and mandibular first permanent molars
3. The **maxillary and mandibular central incisors**

FIGURE 4–41

1. **Enamel hypoplasia** (Turner type) of the mandibular first bicuspid
2. A **microdont** mandibular first bicuspid
3. A **horizontally positioned** developing mandibular **second bicuspid,** which may become horizontally impacted

FIGURE 4–42

Amelogenesis imperfecta, hypoplastic smooth type, affecting both deciduous and permanent teeth. (Note the nearly total absence of enamel.)

FIGURE 4–43

1. It is **gold and acrylic.**
2. This is **calculus.**
3. This represents the **mental foramen.**
Well, did you get these answers? We hoped you would—you know you've seen all this before!

FIGURE 4–44

Once root formation is complete, **the chances of a tooth erupting are markedly reduced.** That is not to say, however, that the tooth cannot be made to erupt with orthodontic intervention. Note the apparent ankylosis of the deciduous second molar.

FIGURE 4–45

1. A **retained deciduous cuspid**
2. An **impacted maxillary permanent cuspid** with advanced or complete root formation
3. **Dens in dente** in the maxillary lateral incisor

FIGURE 4–46

Amelogenesis imperfecta, hypoplastic pitted type

FIGURE 4–47

Peg lateral and **microdont**

FIGURE 4–48

1. **Pulp obliteration.** It is localized in case *A,* generalized in **case *B.***
2. The type in *A* is often secondary to trauma and may eventually require endodontic treatment. Instrumentation of the canal is difficult and sometimes impossible.
3. The type in *B* is usually a result of the physiologic aging process. As such, it is not often associated with any future need for endodontic procedures.

FIGURE 4–49

1. **Extrusion (supraeruption).** The maxillary molars are extruded owing to overeruption.
2. The absence of opposing mandibular teeth causes overeruption of the maxillary teeth. Chronic periodontal disease may also contribute.

FIGURE 4–50

A. 2. **Early caries**
B. 3. **Frank caries**
C. 3. **Frank caries** (deeper than B)
D. 0. **Sound tooth structure**
E. 3. **Frank caries.** (Note that enamel involvement is not obvious.)
F. 0. **Sound tooth structure**

FIGURE 4–51

A. 0. **Sound restoration** (slight overhang)

B. **2. Early caries**

C. **1. Incipient caries** (very close to 2)

FIGURE 4–52

A. **4. Deep recurrent caries**

B. **4. Deep recurrent caries**

C. **3. Frank recurrent caries**

FIGURE 4–53

A. **4. Deep caries**

B. **0.** We interpreted this as **cervical burnout.**

C. **4. Deep occlusal caries.** (Note that the involvement of enamel is rarely seen in occlusal caries.)

FIGURE 4–54

A. **0. Sound enamel**

B. **3. Frank recurrent caries.** (Note the radiopaque **sclerotic dentin** immediately beneath this area showing the typical "arrowhead" appearance with the tip of the arrow pointing to the pulp.)

C. **4. Deep recurrent caries.** (Note that **reparative dentin** is present owing to the altered shape of the pulp horn. Note that it is no more radiopaque than the surrounding dentin, and that it does not show any peculiar configuration.)

D. **0. Sound tooth structure.** We interpreted this as **cervical burnout.**

FIGURE 4–55

A. **3. Frank caries**

B. **2. Early caries**

C. **0. Sound tooth structure**; however, note the **overhang**

D. **4. Deep caries**

E. **0. Sound tooth structure**

F. **0.** The **tooth structure appears sound**; however, **sclerotic dentin** is a radiographic sign of a leaky margin. Therefore, a notation should be made to check this surface carefully clinically.

FIGURE 4–56

Arrow A:

1. **Periapical granuloma; periapical cyst; periapical abscess**

2. **Deep mesial interproximal caries with pulp involvement.** Note that the caries has probably invaded the pulp, but it does not apear to have done so radiographically.

Arrow B:

1. **Periapical granuloma; periapical cyst; periapical abscess**

2. **Deep distal caries**

FIGURE 4–57

Arrow A:

1. **Periapical cyst; periapical granuloma; periapical abscess**

2. Probably a **microscopic pulp exposure** during the preparation of the tooth for the casting

Note: Because of the proximity of the inferior alveolar canal, this patient may experience paresthesia.

FIGURE 4–58

Arrow A:

1. **Periapical cyst; periapical granuloma; periapical abscess**

2. **Deep caries**

Arrow B:

1. **Apical periodontitis**

2. **Deep recurrent caries** due to a defective restoration

FIGURE 4–59

1. **Radiation caries**

2. The **maxillary second bicuspid** (cervical caries)

3. They are thought to be secondary to the xerostomia brought about by radiation atrophy of the major and minor salivary glands within the field of the primary beam. In addition to the alteration in the quantity of the saliva, there appears to be some change in the quality of the remaining saliva that creates a cariogenic environment. Radiation does not appear to have any direct effect on the hard structures of the teeth themselves.

4. a. By proper evaluation of the patient's teeth, periodontium, and attitude prior to radiation therapy.

   b. By immediate extraction of undesirable teeth prior to or early in the course of therapy.

c. By patient education and home-care training, including instruction in the use of dental floss and self-application of topical fluorides.

d. By frequent dental check-ups both in the early months prior to the possible return of some salivary flow and in the long term because of the ever-present threat of developing osteoradionecrosis.

FIGURE 4–60

1. a. **Periapical cyst**
   b. **Periapical granuloma**
   c. **Periapical abscess**
   d. **Periapical cemental dysplasia** in the osteolytic stage

2. **The vitality test.** The fact that a tooth is vital is a strong indication that the lesion represents an early cementoma, which, according to current thinking, requires no further treatment.

FIGURE 4–61

1. In the case of the **mandibular first molar** there are periapical radiolucent lesions associated with an apparently carious tooth. Note also the bifurcation involvement, which may be associated with a high lateral canal. The bone surrounding this tooth is "reactive," a fact that is evidenced by the indistinct trabecular pattern and the more sclerotic appearance of the bone.

2. In the **mandibular second molar** there is the incomplete apexification associated with normal dental development in a twelve year old child.

Note the similarities between the two conditions and the lack of a distinct lamina dura at both apices.

Note also that because of the patient's age the bifurcation involvement would more likely be of pulpal origin than of periodontal origin, though this radiograph alone does not definitively prove this.

FIGURE 4–62

1. A **large mesial carious lesion.** It is interesting to note that in deciduous teeth bifurcation involvement as a sequela to caries is the rule rather than the exception, whereas in permanent teeth it is the excep-

tion rather than the rule. Compare this with Figure 4–61.

2. **Yes**

3. **Turner's enamel hypoplasia**

Well, that's it for the series on caries and the sequelae of caries. But remember: if something in the remaining case presentations looks like caries, don't rule it out, because you know we have a way of repeating things once in a while just to keep you sharp!

FIGURE 4–63

1. **The tip of the nose**
2. **The upper lip** (lower edge)
3. A **fractured incisal** edge of the maxillary left central incisor
4. a. **Accentuated cingulum**
   b. **Dens evaginatus**

FIGURE 4–64

1. **Amalgam overhang** on the mesial of the mandibular first molar
2. The **mandibular second bicuspid,** owing to the bulbous root

FIGURE 4–65

Probably yes, because of the comparatively large pulp chambers whose pulp horns are relatively close to the surface of the teeth

FIGURE 4–66

1. **Macrodontia** of the second bicuspid
2. A **supernumerary root** on the first bicuspid

FIGURE 4–67

Generalized microdontia

FIGURE 4–68

1. a. **Enamel hypoplasia** of the deciduous cuspid, first molar, and second molar teeth
   b. **Congenitally missing** (anodontia) permanent right central and lateral incisors, cuspid, and first and second bicuspids
   c. **Exfoliated or missing** deciduous central and lateral incisors
   d. **Enamel pearls** on deciduous molars

e. Prominent **nutrient canals** in the first molar, cuspid, and incisor areas

2. Hereditary anhidrotic ectodermal dysplasia

FIGURE 4–69

Severe attrition

FIGURE 4–70

1. **"Thistle tube" pulp chamber morphology; pulp stones;** and mild **attrition**
2. **Dentin dysplasia, type II**

FIGURE 4–71

1. **Yes.** He has an avulsed and reimplanted mandibular lateral incisor.
2. **Retrograde amalgam in the avulsed tooth**
3. **External resorption** of the apical two thirds of the root of the mandibular left central incisor, with **ankylosis** of the remaining third. The prognosis for this tooth is further complicated by the presence of calculus and its periodontal implications at the cervix. The large diastemas at the mesial and distal are unusual in this area and may be indicative of flaring of the left lateral incisor.

FIGURE 4–72

1. **Fusion (synodontism)** of the maxillary right deciduous central and lateral incisors
2. Probably **not** the fused deciduous teeth. Rather, the developing supernumerary tooth or odontoma superimposed on the crown of the impacted maxillary right central incisor is the probable cause.

Note that fusion in the primary teeth is sometimes associated with hypodontia of the permanent teeth.

FIGURE 4–73

1. In the **maxillary right central incisor** there is cessation of development, with incomplete root formation and apexification; root fracture; and crown fracture.
2. In the **maxillary left central incisor** apexification appears complete. Therefore, root formation must have been completed and internal resorption subsequently begun. There is also a crown fracture.

3. In the **maxillary left lateral incisor** obliteration of the pulp chamber and root canal is present.

FIGURE 4–74

1. **Painful pulpitis.** Note the thickening of the periodontal membrane space at the apex of the mesial root of the mandibular first molar.
2. Because of **bacterial contamination of the pulp.** Note the microfissure, which is delineated by the well-condensed amalgam that has filled the defect close to the mesial pulp horn.
3. **11½ to 12½ years.** Note the incomplete apexification of the bicuspid and second molar.
4. An **enamel pearl** on the mandibular first molar. Do not confuse this with a pulp stone, which is rarely perfectly circular in shape and rarely below the floor of the pulp chamber. Since endodontic therapy is imminent, this is an important consideration.

FIGURE 4–75

Attrition

FIGURE 4–76

Fusion (synodontism) between the deciduous lateral incisor and a supernumerary deciduous lateral. Fusion is the union between dentin and at least one other dental tissue. This case involves two tooth buds.

Note: The distinction between fusion and gemination is often difficult to establish in a definitive manner by radiographs alone.

FIGURE 4–77

Gemination (schizodontism). In gemination a single tooth attempts to divide into two teeth. The patient has a normal complement of teeth. This condition involves only one tooth bud.

FIGURE 4–78

1. **Hypercementosis.** Note the dentinal outline of the root within the cemental mass.
2. **Paget disease (osteitis deformans)**
3. a. **Periodontal disease**
   b. **Extrusion**

FIGURE 4–79

1. A **dilacerated root** on the maxillary right second bicuspid

2. **Mucous retention phenomenon** of the maxillary sinus adjacent to the apex of the maxillary first molar (differential: maxillary [antral] mucositis)

3. An **erupting fourth molar** (distomolar)

FIGURE 4–80

1. a. The tooth is the **distal abutment** for the fixed bridge.

   b. The tooth appears radiographically to be **ankylosed.**

2. An **amalgam tattoo**

FIGURE 4–81

An incompletely formed **supernumerary root** on the mandibular first permanent molar. (Note the large root canal and wide-open apex.)

FIGURE 4–82

Amelogenesis imperfecta, hypoplastic smooth type

FIGURE 4–83

1. **Dens in dente**
2. **Pulpitis and pulp necrosis**
3. **Shallow pit restoration**
4. **The maxillary lateral incisor**
5. **Yes**

FIGURE 4–84

1. **Dentinogenesis imperfecta**
2. **Yes**
3. These teeth have **susceptibility** to caries about equal to that of normal teeth.
4. **Osteogenesis imperfecta**

FIGURE 4–85

No. This periapical radiolucency actually represents the superior opening of the incisive canal, a normal anatomic landmark. The endodontic procedures were initiated as the result of a fracture of the crown, with a pulp exposure. (Note the fractured crown in the radiograph.)

FIGURE 4–86

1. **Root fracture**

2. **Case A.** Note the large resin restoration, which has weakened the tooth.

3. **Case B.** Note closely the bone that has filled the space between the two segments, and the lack of "reactivity" of the apical fragment.

4. **Case A.** The remaining root structure appears sound and with endodontic treatment would probably support a post and core and crown restoration.

FIGURE 4–87

Impacted maxillary right first, second, and third molars

FIGURE 4–88

Calculus

FIGURE 4–89

Enamel pearls (enamelomas)

FIGURE 4–90

Well, it's simple really. The horizontal angulation was such that the bifurcation of each root became superimposed, producing the **"enamel pearl artifact."** Note the V shape of the periodontal membrane spaces as they criss-cross immediately beneath the artifact. At arrow B there is no criss-crossing of the periodontal membrane space and no artifact!

FIGURE 5-1

1. **Benign.** Notice that the lesion is well delineated by a thin radiopaque line. Malignant lesions tend to be more poorly defined, with more ragged, indistinct borders, but this is not a hard and fast rule.
2. **Residual dentigerous cyst**
3. **Primordial cyst**
4. **Biopsy.** This is mandatory, since dentigerous cysts may be associated with or give rise to a variety of odontogenic neoplasms. Treatment, prognosis, and follow-up are based upon a definitive diagnosis. **The biopsy revealed that this was an ameloblastoma.**

FIGURE 5-2

1. **Traumatic bone cyst.** The age of the patient and history of trauma are helpful hints. Radiographically, the lesion is unilocular and is well delineated, with a sclerotic border at its superior portion. Note that the lesion appears to be "squeezing up" between the bicuspids, with minimal displacement of the roots. Though the lamina dura is often intact, in this case there appears to be some destruction.
2. **Pulp test** (electrical, hot, cold, percussion)
3. **Surgical exploration.** Usually an empty cavity with no discernible lining is found.
4. **Lateral periodontal cyst, primordial cyst of a supernumerary tooth, central giant cell granuloma,** and **ameloblastic fibroma.** The last two lesions are especially noteworthy, since they also tend to occur in this age group and in this location.

FIGURE 5-3

1. **Benign.** The mandibular canal appears to be expanded inferiorly almost to the inferior border of the mandible and superiorly to a level above the mylohyoid ridge. Notice that the cortical bone lining the canal is completely intact.
2. a. **Anatomic variation.** This is unlikely, since you would not expect a paresthesia to be associated with a normal canal and since upon further examination the right mandibular canal was normal in size.
   b. **Lingual mandibular salivary gland depression.** This is unlikely, since this "lesion," though mainly found in this area, is usually below the canal. The appearance in the radiograph of the salivary gland depression is pathognomonic.
   c. **Metastatic disease.** This is possible, since paresthesia is an associated (and ominous) sign. However, metastatic disease would not be so well delineated.
   d. **Adenoid cystic carcinoma.** This is possible, since the neoplasm produces paresthesia by perineural invasion. This, however, usually occurs in soft tissue containing salivary gland parenchyma rather than in central bone.
   e. **Benign neural lesion.** This is most likely, and three good choices would be neurilemmoma, neurofibroma, and traumatic neuroma.
   f. **Vascular lesion.** Always consider a vascular lesion in the jaws, especially at this anatomic location.

FIGURE 5-4

1. **Lingual mandibular salivary gland depression**
2. Typically, such salivary gland depressions appear as a **round, ovoid,** or **triangular radiolucency** that is located in the **posterior** portion of the body of the mandible, **below the mandibular canal** and **above the inferior cortex.** The depression may encroach upon the mandibular canal and/or the inferior cortex.

FIGURE 5-5

1. **Supernumerary tooth bud** and **developing odontoma**
2. **Lateral periodontal cyst**
3. **Retained deciduous root tip, sialolith, torus mandibularis,** and **buccal surface exostosis**

FIGURE 5-6

1. It appears to be a **compound odontoma** associated with supernumerary and impacted mandibular bicuspids.

2. **Yes. This is done in order to rule out associated pathologic conditions** such as ameloblastoma or odontogenic keratocyst, which would definitely increase the possibility of recurrence, and to confirm definitively the clinical and radiographic data.

FIGURE 5-7

Lingual mandibular tori

FIGURE 5-8

1. The patient is probably **11½ to 12 years old** (possibly as young as 10½ or as old as 13). Notice the open apices of the mandibular second premolar and second molar.

2. Mesial and distal **retained root tips** of the primary second molar

3. **No.** Sometimes the second bicuspid erupts without complete resorption of the root tips of the primary molar. This phenomenon is sometimes seen in all four quadrants of a single patient's dentition.

FIGURE 5-9

1. It may have been caused by a **primordial cyst** of a supernumerary tooth or by the **epithelial rests of Malassez,** which undergo cystic transformation.

2. **Yes,** as high as 50 per cent within five years when it is of the odontogenic keratocyst type

FIGURE 5-10

1. **Sialolith, calcified lymph node, osteoma, calcified thrombus,** or **dystrophic calcification** in a soft tissue lesion such as a hemangioma. Do not look at the answer to part 2. That's not fair.

   2. a. By taking an **occlusal view** radiograph. This would determine whether the radiopacity is located buccal or lingual to the body of the mandible.

      b. If it is not located bucally, the osteotoma would be a likely choice. It

could be confirmed by palpating the inferior border of the mandible and by biopsy.

      c. If this opacity is medial to the body of the mandible, a sialogram would help to determine whether it represents a sialolith or a calcified submaxillary lymph node.

      d. If the opacity is lateral to the body of the mandible, a calcified thrombus might be the cause. Confirm this diagnosis by biopsy.

      e. In the case of the hemangioma, the finding of soft tissue discoloration is significant. Biopsy may be contraindicated.

Note: In this case, the occlusal view demonstrated that the opacity was medial to the mandible. The sialogram showed delayed emptying time and pooling of the radiopaque contrast material proximal to the stone. The ducts showed signs of sialodochitis, which often accompanies salivary calculi. **Final diagnosis: sialolith in the right Wharton duct and secondary sialodochitis of the right submaxillary gland.**

FIGURE 5-11

   1. a. **Periodontitis**
      b. **Scleroderma**
      c. **Early osteosarcoma or fibrosarcoma**
      d. **Normal anatomic variation**
      e. **Traumatic occlusion**

2. Our most likely choice in this case is a **normal anatomic variation** or **traumatic occlusion.**

Periodontal disease is unlikely since the prominent lamina dura is intact; also, the height of the alveolar crest appears normal.

Scleroderma is unlikely since the widened PDM space is not generalized.

Early osteosarcoma is a possibility. The patient's age, sex, and history of pain would also be helpful in establishing this diagnosis. Clinical observation of abnormally large wear facets and tooth mobility would be helpful.

   3. a. **Normal anatomic variation**
      b. **Traumatic occlusion**
      c. **Osteopetrosis**

FIGURE 5–12

1. **Retained root tip**
2. a. In the **cuspid region** of the maxilla
   b. **Inverted "Y"**
3. **The nasolabial fold**

FIGURE 5–13

1. **Cherubism**
2. **Yes,** but not necessarily from a single periapical film. However, bilateral multilocular expansile lesions involving the entire mandible or (sometimes) the maxilla or both may be considered pathognomonic signs of cherubism. Characteristically, there is thinning of the cortical plates and, paradoxically, no tendency for pathologic fracture. Also, delayed eruption and malformation of the permanent teeth are sometimes seen.

FIGURE 5–14

1. It may be **normal.** This pattern is often seen in normal persons, especially between the roots of a mandibular first molar.
2. It may represent **sickle cell anemia.** This possibility should be investigated until it can be confirmed or ruled out. Sickle cell anemia is known to cause alterations of the trabecular pattern as the marrow spaces become enlarged during the pathogenesis of the disease. One of these alterations of the trabecular pattern is referred to as the "step ladder" effect. Since this pattern is seen in this radiograph, the possibility of this disease must be investigated.

FIGURE 5–15

1. **Focal osteoporotic bone marrow defect of the jaw**
2. By **biopsy**

Note: The fibrous healing defect might be a possibility, but this is usually more radiolucent and more well defined and is often located in the maxillary bicuspid and anterior areas.

The osteoporotic bone marrow defect is often located in the mandibular molar region. It is seen most often in middle aged women. In the pathogenesis of this lesion, the lamina dura of the socket disappears, but the crestal bone is intact. The area remains relatively more radiolucent and often contains fine, sparse trabeculae.

FIGURE 5–16

1. As **soon as possible after dialysis**
2. **Socket sclerosis**
3. **Persistence of the lamina dura** and **filling of the socket area with sclerotic bone,** beginning at the base of the socket and proceeding toward the crest of the ridge but **not extending beyond the confines of the socket**
4. **Renal disease** and **intestinal malabsorption disorders**
5. **Yes.** Note that the roof has a bulbous shape—that is, the apex is wider than the cervical portion.

FIGURE 5–17

1. It is a **periapical abscess, periapical cyst,** or **periapical granuloma**
2. The **mental foramen**
3. a. The mandibular first bicuspid has a **dilacerated root.**
   b. The first bicuspid probably has **two roots.** The signs of this are abrupt narrowing of the root canal space and "double" periodontal membrane space.
   c. There also appears to be **some obliteration of the root canal space.**

FIGURE 5–18

It represents **chronic focal sclerosing osteomyelitis** (condensing osteitis). Note the deep restoration and the lack of continuity of the lamina dura around the apex of the tooth.

These last two cases demonstrate two different responses of alveolar bone to the same stimulus. In one case (Fig. 5–17) the periapical infection resulted in lysis of bone, while in the other case (this figure) there was production of bone.

FIGURE 5–19

1. **Osteosclerosis** (sclerotic bone)
2. **Calcified submaxillary lymph node**
3. **Sialolith**
4. **Enostosis or exostosis**
5. **Osteoma**

Note: The mature cementoma is not likely because of the lack of a radiolucent line demarcating the lesion.

Now remember, sclerotic bone appears identical to condensing osteitis. In the latter case the tooth may show some sign of pulpitis. The distinction between these two painless conditions is important because sclerotic bone requires no treatment while condensing osteitis requires management, usually pulp therapy.

FIGURE 5–20

1. **Periapical cemental dysplasia** in the osteolytic phase. No treatment is necessary.
2. **Chronic diffuse sclerosing osteomyelitis** when multiple mature cementomas are present. A single periapical lesion in the radiolucent stage mimics a periapical lesion of pulpal origin—that is to say, a **periapical abscess, cyst, or granuloma.**

FIGURE 5–21

1. **Periapical cyst**
2. **Periapical granuloma**
3. **Periapical abscess**

Note: This lesion represents one of two possible periapical reactions when the floor of the maxillary sinus is involved. The reaction here is a case of **"periapical halo formation"** and is not necessarily a cyst. It represents a deposition of reactive bone bulging into the maxillary sinus. The other reaction is known as **periapical mucositis.**

FIGURE 5–22

1. **Mucous retention cyst of the maxillary sinus**
2. **Periapical mucositis.** Remember, the only difference between a mucous retention cyst of the maxillary sinus and periapical mucositis is that in the latter case the cause is a pulpally involved tooth.
3. **The distinction between these two conditions is important because the mucous retention cyst requires no treatment, whereas periapical mucositis requires management, usually pulp therapy.**

FIGURE 5–23

1. a. **Periapical cyst**
   b. **Periapical granuloma**
   c. **Periapical abscess**

d. **Superior foramen of the incisive canal**
e. **Incisive canal cyst**
f. **Primordial cyst of a mesiodens**
2. Note the obliteration of the root canal space. This is an indication of a history of chronic painless pulpitis. The presence of the temporary filling material in the central portion of the crown indicates that an attempt was made to extirpate the pulp. It may be further supposed that this procedure was carried out because the tooth was found to be nonvital. The tooth appears to have been restored very conservatively, and the most likely reason for the development of the periapical lesion was the subsequent development of an anachoretic pulpitis and its sequelae. Anachoretic pulpitis often develops in teeth that have been devitalized by trauma.

FIGURE 5–24

1. a. **Residual dentigerous cyst**
   b. **Incisive canal cyst**
   c. **Globulomaxillary cyst**
   d. **Odontogenic adenomatoid tumor**
   e. **Fibrous healing defect**
2. The **palatoglossal air space,** caused when the patient fails to place the tongue firmly against the palate as in swallowing

Note: The lesion in this case was a **residual dentigerous cyst.**

FIGURE 5–25

Compound fracture of the mandible
Any questions?

FIGURE 5–26

1. **Cervical burn-out**
2. a. **Deep caries** with radiographic encroachment upon the pulp space
   b. **Obliteration of the** apical portion of the **root canal space Hypercementosis**
   c. **Loss of** a large area of the **apical lamina dura and/or sinus floor Periapical mucositis**

Did you get it? You knew this was coming!

FIGURE 5–27

1. a. **Ameloblastoma**
   b. **Odontogenic myxoma**

c. **Odontogenic keratocyst**
d. **Central giant cell granuloma**
2. The **ameloblastoma** is the best choice. The **odontogenic myxoma** generally has much finer striations or locules; the **odontogenic keratocyst** is an excellent possibility, but the locules are rarely this well defined (instead they tend to produce more of the scalloping around the edges of the cyst rather than the central part); the **central giant cell granuloma** rarely extends more posteriorly than the bicuspids.

FIGURE 5–28

1. **Black**
2. **Over 40 years of age**
3. **Female**
4. **Yes**
5. **Periapical cemental dysplasia** (cementoma). This condition is in the osteolytic stage in patient *A,* the cementoblastic stage in patient *B,* and the mature stage in patient *C.*

Note: In the mature stage the cementoma is often crescent-shaped, with the apex of the tooth fitting into the concave surface. The involved apex is usually clearly visible and the lesion is surrounded by a radiolucent outline. See radiograph C.

FIGURE 5–29

1. It is a **benign cementoblastoma.** Note the following radiographic features:
    a. Radiopacity is obliterating the root apex.
    b. The early lesion appears to be delineated by an intact periodontal membrane space in some areas.
    c. The mature lesion is well delineated by a peripheral radiolucent area.
    d. The tooth appears otherwise normal radiographically.
2. **Yes**
3. **Excision.** This may involve removal of the tooth. These lesions, although benign, are considered to have excessive growth potential.

Note: The relatively opaque alveolar bone in the upper half of the radiograph probably represents a focal sclerosing osteomyelitis secondary to the periodontal disease that is present.

FIGURE 5–30

This one is **periapical cemental dysplasia** (cementoma).

FIGURE 5–31

The probable reason for this extraction is **painful pulpitis** (toothache). This may be the cause of the focal sclerosing osteomyelitis present at the apical portion of the distal socket. Notice the intact lamina dura lining most of the remaining socket areas, which indicates a previously healthy periodontal status of the tooth.

Notice a slight interruption of the lamina dura at the apical portion of the mesial socket, indicating an apical periodontitis that has led to a localized breakdown of the lamina dura lining the socket. The tooth was extracted before any further periapical pathologic condition could develop.

It is interesting to note that the distal apex appears to have an associated chronic condition, which is often painless, whereas the mesial apex was associated with an early acute reaction, which is often painful.

Note: This should not be interpreted as the beginning of **socket sclerosis,** which usually does not extend beyond the confines of the original socket.

FIGURE 5–32

Median maxillary anterior alveolar cleft

FIGURE 5–33

1. **Cleft palate**
2. **Peg lateral incisor**
3. The **ala of the nose**

FIGURE 5–34

Developmental lingual mandibular salivary gland depression
Note: When this "lesion" occurs in the anterior area it is not specific or definitive in appearance. The borders are often not well delineated and it may mimic other pathologic conditions.

FIGURE 5–35

Distal mandibular hyperostosis (pseudohyperostosis)

Comment: This condition is an apparent increase in height of the alveolar bone seen on the distal of the last molar in the mandibular arch. This may involve the first, second, or third molar. There are two situations in which this condition may be noted:

1. the situation in which a molar distal to the tooth in question has been extracted and the alveolar bone level immediately distal to the remaining molar remains high relative to the remainder of the ridge, and

2. that in which the molar in question is tilted to the mesial. A pseudopocket is noted on the mesial, whereas on the distal or tension side an apparent "build-up" of alveolar bone is noted.

FIGURE 5–36

1. **Enlarged genial tubercles**
2. **Possibly.** Note that the patient is edentulous. As the ridge resorbs, the denture flange would tend to traumatize this area.

FIGURE 5–37

1. **Chin tilted too high.** Note the flat occlusal plane and the condyles very close to the right and left edges of the film.
2. **Palatoglossal air space.** This is caused when the patient fails to hold the tongue against the palate.
   3. a. **Dentigerous** (follicular) **cyst**
      b. **Odontogenic keratocyst,** dentigerous subtype
      c. **Ameloblastoma**
      d. **Gorlin cyst**
      e. **Ameloblastic fibroma**

Note: This could be an odontogenic keratocyst due to its moderate size, evidence of expansion at the crest of the ridge, cloudy lumen, and possible displacement of the third molar. Since mural ameloblastomas arise from dentigerous cysts, any larger dentigerous cyst should be suspected to have undergone this change.

The **keratinizing and calcifying epithelial odontogenic** (Gorlin) **cyst** is associated with an unerupted tooth in 20% of cases, can occur at any age or location, and may have calcified material in the lumen.

The **ameloblastic fibroma** almost always occurs in association with an un-erupted or impacted tooth. Male patients *are* subject to this lesion—*and* at the location shown in the figure—but they are usually a bit younger than 19 (the age of the patient in this case) when the ameloblastic fibroma arises.

(This was in fact a **dentigerous cyst** and this is a typical example of this cyst.)

4. **Dentigerous cyst**

FIGURE 5–38

1. First, did you recognize that the circular radiopaque structure in the center of the lesion is the **tip of the nose?** As for the lesion itself, possible diagnoses include:
   a. **Incisive canal cyst** (nasopalatine duct cyst)
   b. **Primordial cyst** of a mesiodens
   c. **Residual cyst** (from a central incisor)
   d. **Gorlin cyst**
   e. **Odontogenic keratocyst**

Note: You may not have realized that **odontogenic keratocysts in the maxilla** tend to be smaller, solitary, and in the anterior region.

2. **Incisive canal cyst**

FIGURE 5–39

1. **Pericoronitis.** Notice the poorly defined radiolucency seen around the distal portion of the crown of the third molar; it is often seen in this condition.

2. **No.** The roots now appear to be fully formed; thus the tooth's eruptive potential is greatly diminished. Notice also that the tooth is vertically impacted with the crown in slight distoversion.

FIGURE 5–40

1. a. **Popcorn kernel** or other foreign body
   b. **Juvenile periodontitis** (periodontosis)
   c. **Eosinophilic granuloma**
   d. **Diabetes mellitus**
   e. **Papillon-Lefèvre syndrome**
   f. **Chédiak-Higashi syndrome**
   g. **Neutropenia**

2. **Juvenile periodontitis.** The age, sex, and race of the patient and the location of

the lesions are classic. Note also what appears to be the beginning of bone loss on the distal of the cuspid. This area is also commonly affected. Note the lack of calculus.

FIGURE 5-41

Eruption cyst

FIGURE 5-42

Eruption sequestrum

FIGURE 5-43

Hyperostosis (under the bridge pontic)

FIGURE 5-44

Torus palatinus. In radiograph A you can almost make out concentric growth rings indicative of the lesion's growth; in radiograph B the torus is multi-lobed.

FIGURE 5-45

1. **Attrition**
2. Moderate **pulpal obliteration**
3. **Cementoma** (lower right central incisor)
4. **Bilateral** multi-lobed **mandibular lingual tori**
5. From the shape of the radiolucency, it seems that the distal of the **right lateral incisor has been restored.**

FIGURE 5-46

1. **Osteoma** arising from the wall of the maxillary antrum
2. **Antrolith**
3. **Root tip**
4. **Sialolith** near the parotid papilla. This is unlikely, since the parotid papilla is usually adjacent to the maxillary first molar, which in this radiograph would be near the malar process.
5. **Soft tissue calcification** in the buccal mucosa

FIGURE 5-47

This is often referred to as a **"cloudy sinus"** and in this case represents an **antral mucositis** probably associated with the carious first and second molars.

Note: Infected teeth are not always the cause of a cloudy sinus. The most common cause of a cloudy sinus is chronic sinusitis. Paradoxically, this latter condition may often be associated with odontalgia, and the dental practitioner is often called upon to rule out the teeth as the cause of the patient's discomfort. The presence of fluid in the maxillary sinus may be reconfirmed by taking the Waters' sinus radiographic view and by transillumination of the sinus.

FIGURE 5-48

1. **The lesion in radiograph B**
2. a. The lesion is about 2 cm in diameter in both radiograph A and radiograph B.
   b. With the lesion at the stage shown in radiograph A, radiopaque material is obliterating root apices; at the stage shown in radiograph B, radiopaque material almost obliterates root apices.
   c. At the stage shown in A, there is a wide band of radiolucent material surrounding the radiopaque core, signifying an early lesion; at the stage shown in B, there is a thin but distinct band of radiolucent material surrounding the radiopaque core, signifying a mature lesion.
   d. The tooth affected in radiograph A—mandibular molar—is the most common site of the lesion; the tooth affected in radiograph B—mandibular second molar—is a common location.
   e. The tooth appears vital radiographically in both A and B.
   f. The tooth in A appears to be extruded due to the lesion (note, though, that this is an unusual finding and that the extrusion may be due to the absence of the maxillary tooth); in B there is no tooth displacement by the lesion (a usual finding).
3. **Benign cementoblastoma**
4. **Removal of the lesion**—and, usually, of the tooth as well, as the two are rarely separable

Note: You may have noticed that both teeth have **pulp stones,** an incidental finding, but unusual for the age of these patients.

FIGURE 5-49

1. **Osteosclerosis** (sclerotic bone)

Well, we hoped you'd get this. Note that the tooth is vital and that there is **no radiolucent line** delineating the sclerotic bone from the surrounding normal bone. Incidentally, if you said osteoma you would be partly right, as osteoma, exostosis, enostosis, osteosclerosis, and torus may all be histologically identical, and the distinction is made solely upon the clinical and radiographic presentation.

2. Patients of Mexican-American ancestry sometimes present with the **shovel-shaped incisor syndrome**. The two main features of this syndrome are (1) blunted and shortened or tapered roots, particularly those of the mandibular bicuspids, and (2) prominent marginal ridges on the maxillary incisors. In this case you will note the shortening and blunting of the mandibular second premolar and the maxillary first premolar. Thus it was our impression that the mandibular second bicuspid was not being resorbed by the radiopaque lesion; this is consistent with the behavior of osteosclerosis.

FIGURE 5-50

1. **Developing odontoma**
2. **Yes**
3. **No.** The histologic diagnosis may confirm several other alternatives. First, the lesion may not be an odontoma as such but rather a dentinoma or a cementifying or ossifying odontogenic lesion. Second, the pathologic report may confirm that this is an odontoma that is associated with other pathologic findings such as an ameloblastoma or even a malignant lesion. All of these possibilities will affect the prognosis, additional treatment, and follow-up of the patient.

By the way . . . . You will note that this lesion is well demarcated by a radiolucent line. This is a constant feature of all odontomas, especially developing odontomas. Such a line is also a feature of an inverted developing supernumerary tooth, as well as other radiopaque lesions. Thus, one thing the lesion in this figure *is not* is osteosclerosis; nor can it be a mandibular torus. Are you starting to catch on?

FIGURE 5-51

1. a. **Central cementifying fibroma**
   b. **Central ossifying fibroma**
   c. **Central cemento-ossifying fibroma**
   d. **Benign cementoblastoma**
   e. **Complex odontoma**
2. **Any one of the first three choices** listed above, as they are all related and have similar characteristics.

Note: This lesion was in fact a **central cementifying fibroma**. A prominent feature is its ball-like growth pattern with a resultant expansion of the buccal and lingual cortical plates and displacement of adjacent teeth. The apparent root resorption in this case is a bit unusual. The lesion is well delineated from the surrounding bone.

FIGURE 5-52

Diagnostic possibilities:
   a. **Calcifying epithelial odontogenic tumor of Pindborg (CEOT)**
   b. **Central cementifying, ossifying, or cemento-ossifying fibroma**
   c. **Keratinizing and calcifying odontogenic cyst (KCOC)**
   d. **Complex odontoma**
   e. **Ameloblastic odontoma**
   f. **Fibrous dysplasia**

Note: This was a **Pindborg tumor.** Some features of this tumor are: its association with impaction of a tooth that is not usually impacted; radiopaque flecks resembling "driven snow"; expansion, often of the buccal cortical plate; and poor delineation from surrounding bone.

FIGURE 5-53

Complex odontoma. Remember, complex odontomas tend to be posterior in either jaw, while compound odontomas tend to be located in the maxilla, anterior to the first molar.

Well, don't get discouraged! This would be a good time to take a break . . . . There's more to come!

FIGURE 5–54

Mucous retention cyst of the maxillary sinus

FIGURE 5–55

1. **Nutrient canals**
2. **Calculus**
3. **Periodontal disease**

FIGURE 5–56

Fibrous healing defect

FIGURE 5–57

Exostosis or **osteoma** is the diagnosis. **Excision** in order to avoid interference with the mandibular dentures is the treatment. **Biopsy** is mandatory for confirmation of the diagnosis.

FIGURE 5–58

1. It is a circumscribed radiopacity surrounding the root and periapical areas of the mandibular first and second molars and extending into the edentulous third molar area. The bone has a **"ground glass"** appearance, and there is **no distinct lamina dura** in this area.
    2. a. **Fibrous dysplasia**
       b. **Hyperparathyroidism**
       c. **Paget disease**
       d. **Dominant cranio-metaphyseal dysplasia**
    3. **Fibrous dysplasia**

FIGURE 5–59

Secondary hyperparathyroidism. This condition is produced as a result of increased renal excretion of calcium, which results in decreased serum levels of calcium. This stimulates production of parathyroid hormone, which results in increased serum calcium. Note that the increased urinary secretion of calcium is a sequela of the chronic renal disease and that, unlike the elevated serum Ca levels seen in primary hyperparathyroidism, the serum Ca levels seen in secondary hyperparathyroidism are often normal to high normal.

Note the **"ground glass"** trabecular pattern and the generalized loss of the lamina dura. Note also that the more advanced giant cell lesion on the patient's right side (radiograph *A*) is producing root resorption and extrusion of the molar.

FIGURE 5–60

1. **Paget disease**
2. a. **Loss of the lamina dura**
   b. **Hypercementosis**
   c. **Cotton wool** appearance of the alveolar bone
3. **Chronic diffuse sclerosing osteomyelitis**

Note: The taking of a head plate might help in the radiographic evaluation.

FIGURE 5–61

1. a. **Multiple cementomas**
   b. **Chronic diffuse sclerosing osteomyelitis** (florid osseous dysplasia)
   c. **Paget disease**
2. **Chronic diffuse sclerosing osteomyelitis**
3. **None** (as long as the patient remains asymptomatic)

FIGURE 5–62

Chronic osteomyelitis of the left mandible

FIGURE 5–63

1. a. **Garré's osteomyelitis**
   b. **Ewing's sarcoma**
   c. **Osteogenic sarcoma**
   d. **Chondrosarcoma**
2. **Garré's osteomyelitis**
3. **Antibiotics.** Penicillin is still the drug of choice in most cases. The antibiotics should be continued for one to two weeks. The swelling may persist for several more weeks, even months. Resolution usually occurs within three to six months. Note that the offending tooth has been extracted.

FIGURE 5–64

1. **Dentigerous** (follicular)
2. a. **Primordial**
   b. **Lateral periodontal**
   c. **Idiopathic**
   d. **OKC of the jaw occurring in basal cell nevus syndrome**
   e. **Periapical.** (Recent reports indi-

cate that some periapical cysts may be OKC's.)

3. a. **Large size**
   b. **Scalloped border,** tending toward multilocularity
   c. **Expansion**
   d. **Displacement** of unerupted or developing teeth
   e. **Multiple cysts** (in some cases)
   f. **Perforation** of the cortical plate
   g. **Cloudy lumen** (milky-way lumen)
4. **Basal cell nevus syndrome**
   a. **Basal cell nevi** on the skin
   b. **Odontogenic keratocysts** in the jaws
   c. **Bifid ribs** and other skeletal deformities
5. **Recurrence.** The recurrence rate of OKC's is 50 per cent within 3 to 5 years.

Note: Recurrences are said to be more likely when the odontogenic keratocysts: (1) occur as part of the basal cell nevus syndrome; (2) are large and multilocular and perforate into soft tissue; and (3) are difficult to surgically separate from the bone and tend to require removal in multiple segments.

FIGURE 5–65

1. **Hyoid bone.** The body appears to be superimposed on the inferior border of the mandible, and the tips of the greater horns are superimposed on the lesion.
2. a. **Sialolith**
   b. **Calcified lymph node**
   c. **Phlebolith**
   d. **Soft tissue osteoma**
   Note: This was a **calcified lymph node.**

FIGURE 5–66

1. Place a No. 2 intraoral film with the plain side against the buccal mucosa. Have the patient hold the film with his index finger. Decrease exposure factors so as not to "burn out" the poorly calcified lesions. Usually the kV is reduced to about 60 and the mAs factor is reduced by 50 per cent.
2. a. **Osteoma cutis.** The density is correct, and the round, smooth outline is typical.
   b. **Miliary osteomas.** These are often less dense and less well defined; usually there is a radiolucent center that produces a characteristic doughnut-like lesion. When these osteomas occur, they are present in greater numbers than seen here.
   c. **Phleboliths.** The density is correct; however, a vascular lesion is usually present, and characteristically there is a radiolucent component—usually in the center and sometimes occurring as several rings of radiolucent (and radiopaque) material.
   d. **Cysticercosis.** The density is correct; however, one would expect these to be more ovoid in shape, somewhat resembling large grains of rice.
   e. **Calcified acne or smallpox scars.** These lesions are usually not so radiopaque; nor are they so well defined at their periphery—an irregular outline is much more likely. (Also, of course, clinical evidence of the scars is present on the skin.)

Note: We are sorry to report that we never determined the nature of these lesions.

FIGURE 5–67

If you said **buccal mucosa,** you're absolutely right. The film *B* is a view of the soft tissue of the adjacent buccal mucosa. The patient had no history of trauma other than the extraction of some deciduous teeth that had been previously restored.

FIGURE 5–68

A history would obviously be of benefit. This could possibly represent a **large amalgam tattoo** in the maxillary tuberosity, as well as **some other metallic object** in the maxillary sinus. **In actuality,** the patient revealed that she had shot a .32 caliber revolver into a sink. The **bullet** ricocheted back and struck her in the face. The radiograph shows that the bullet entered at the maxillary tuberosity, leaving many fragments behind as it finally lodged in the maxillary antrum.

FIGURE 5–69

1. **Anterior tubercles of C-1** (atlas)
2. **Patient positioned too far forward** in the machine
3. **Palatoglossal air space,** caused when the patient fails to hold the tongue against the palate
4. **Osteoporosis**
5. **High calcium intake,** supplemented with **strontium** and/or **sodium fluoride**

Note: Osteoporosis is now thought to be caused by a long-term negative calcium balance. The condition responds to calcium therapy. The strontium and fluoride help to maintain the bone density in affected patients.

FIGURE 5–70

1. a. **Central giant cell granuloma**
   b. **Brown tumor of hyperparathyroidism**
   c. **Aneurysmal bone cyst**
   d. **Eosinophilic granuloma**
   e. **Central vascular lesions** (hemangioma)
   f. **Malignancy,** such as primary intraalveolar carcinoma or metastatic carcinoma
2. **Central giant cell granuloma.** The **big clue** was the serum calcium. Evaluation of serum calcium is done to rule out hyperparathyroidism when a histologic diagnosis of central giant cell granuloma is received.

FIGURE 5–71

Periodontal disease; gingival carcinoma; eosinophilic granuloma; metastatic carcinoma

Note: This case turned out to be advanced periodontal disease.

FIGURE 5–72

In the mandibular left first molar, caries is present. Alloy restoration would be the obvious choice for treatment. There **appears,** however, to be an **early** benign cementoblastoma associated with the apex of the distal root. Removal of the lesion and, consequently, of the tooth is recommended. This is because the lesion may achieve a large size and it is generally impossible to separate the lesion from the tooth surgically.

Note: The differential diagnosis would include hypercementosis. However, it must be remembered that hypercementosis is rare in this age group, while the benign cementoblastoma does occur at this age and the mandibular first molar is the most common location. A short period of observation might be in order to see if a more typical lesion develops.

FIGURE 5–73

1. **Mandibular molar area.** The clue here is the internal oblique ridge seen on the left of the radiograph.
2. a. **Periapical cemental dysplasia** (cementoma)
   b. **Chronic diffuse sclerosing osteomyelitis**
   c. **Retained root tips**
   d. **Osteoma**
   e. **Osteoid osteoma**
   f. **Sclerotic bone**
3. Using the radiograph alone, this is a difficult question. The "target-like" appearance of the lesions with radiopaque centers, along with the history, strongly suggests **periapical cemental dysplasia** in the mature stage. Chronic diffuse sclerosing osteomyelitis is possible, however, and has a predilection for middle-aged blacks. It has been suggested that these two conditions may in fact be the same.

The osteoma and bone scar are not usually delineated by a circumscribed radiolucent area.

FIGURE 5–74

1. The **maxillary right anterior region**
2. The **maxillary right permanent cuspid**
3. **Follicular cyst** (dentigerous cyst)
4. **Adenomatoid odontogenic tumor** (adenoameloblastoma)
5. The **right nasal fossa**

FIGURE 5–75

1. **Complex** in radiograph *A*
2. **Compound** in radiograph *B*

Well, we hoped you'd get that as the finale for this section!

SECTION 6

FIGURE 6–1

1. An **enameloma** (enamel pearl)
2. **Palatally**

It should be noted that radiograph 6–1A was taken in the usual, prescribed manner. Figure 6–1B was taken with the cone directed toward the anterior of the arch. The enamel pearl appears to have moved or shifted toward the distal or opposite to the direction of flow of the x-ray beam.

FIGURE 6–2

The impacted third molar appears to have shifted toward the anterior of the arch, since it overlaps the second molar. You are correct if you said it is located slightly **buccal** to the second molar.

FIGURE 6–3

There is an extra root on the first molar. It's **located buccally** because it has moved to the anterior with the flow of the beam.

FIGURE 6–4

Remember the rule? If the object moves in the same direction as the flow of the x-ray beam, the object is buccally located. In this case it did, so it is **buccal.**

FIGURE 6–5

We gave you the answer when we said the small silver alloy moved toward the source of radiation, not away from it. **"Lingually"** is the answer.

FIGURE 6–6

It is **lingual,** and we're sure you know the reason why.

FIGURE 6–7

Use the SLOB rule. As you gaze from the patient's left to right, the crown of the tooth moves from being superimposed on the left central to the right central. Can you see that? Therefore, the tooth moved in the same direction as your gaze, meaning it is on the **lingual (palatal).** Now if you reverse the process and gaze from right to left, you will arrive at the same conclusion.

FIGURE 6–8

Once again, look on the patient's left side; the B-B is located between the central incisors. Now gaze to the patient's right and the B-B moves more toward the patient's right, as it is now superimposed on the right central incisor. Did you say **lingual**? Well, you're right. In fact, a lateral head film with the mouth open revealed that the B-B was lodged in the tongue!

FIGURE 6–9

Compare the size of the impacted canine to the contralateral erupted canine. It definitely appears larger, or magnified. It is therefore located toward the **palatal side!**

Well, that's it. Now you're ready for the Review Questions for National and State Board Examinations in Section 7. Good luck!

SECTION 7

FIGURE 7–1

C. **Dilaceration**

FIGURE 7–2

A. **Attrition**

FIGURE 7–3

D. **Enameloma** (enamel pearl)

FIGURE 7–4

D. **Tongue shadow**

FIGURE 7–5

B. **Amelogenesis imperfecta**

FIGURE 7–6

1. C. **Rieger's syndrome,** due to the

possibility of congenital cataracts, the detection and management of which can help prevent blindness in affected children.

2. B. **Dental papilla**

FIGURE 7–7

D. **All of the above**

FIGURE 7–8

1. A. **Diastema.** Note that the primate space occurs only in the primary dentition.
2. A. **Lateral fossa**

FIGURE 7–9

B. **It's a lateral periodontal cyst, but I need to know if it's an odontogenic keratocyst subtype** (because there is a good chance of recurrence and I need to rule out the basal cell nevus syndrome if it is an odontogenic keratocyst subtype).

FIGURE 7–10

1. A. **Patient too far forward**
2. D. **Soft tissue outline of the nose**
3. B. **Ghost image of the hyoid bone**

FIGURE 7–11

A. **Renal disease**
B. **Intestinal malabsorption problems**

FIGURE 7–12

Radiograph A:
   A. **Incisive canal** or **incisive foramen**
Radiograph B:
   B. **Incisive canal cyst.** Note that the appearance of a radiopaque outline is a sure sign of cystic transformation within the incisive canal.

FIGURE 7–13

1. D. **Migration**
2. D. **Palatoglossal air space** due to tongue malpositioning

FIGURE 7–14

1. C. **Sinus recess**
2. A. **Excessive positive vertical angulation. Note:** The signs of this are dimensional distortion—i.e.,

foreshortening of the buccal roots and elongation of the palatal roots—and superimposition of the zygomatic arch on the molars.

FIGURE 7–15

B. **Dentin dysplasia,** type I

FIGURE 7–16

1. A. **Osteosclerosis**

FIGURE 7–17

1. A. **Incisive foramen**
2. C. **Palatal**–notice that the radiolucency is moving in the same direction as the cone tip.
3. A. **Previous orthodontic treatment**

FIGURE 7–18

C. **Developmental lingual mandibular salivary gland depression, posterior variant.**

FIGURE 7–19

B. **Toothbrush abrasion**

FIGURE 7–20

B. **Gemination**

FIGURE 7–21

C. **Palatal.** Note the obvious magnification of the maxillary left canine.

FIGURE 7–22

1. A. **Chin too high**
   D. **Partial denture left in**
   E. **Cotton roll or bite guide not used**
Note that the teeth are in occlusion
2. **Central giant cell granuloma.** Note that the serum calcium studies are done to rule out hyperparathyroidism when a histologic diagnosis of central giant cell granuloma is made. This lesion and the history are typical. Note that root resorption, crossing the midline, and location anterior to the first molars are all typical of this lesion.

FIGURE 7–23

A   **Nasolabial fold**
B   **Lateral wall of nasal fossa**

C **Inferior meatus**
D **Inferior turbinate**
E **Soft tissue of nose**
F **Fibrous healing defect**
G **Gutta-percha**
H **Radiopaque anterior restorative material**

There are no matches for the terms superior foramen of incisive canal and periapical abscess.

FIGURE 7–24

A **Sclerotic dentin**
B **Cervical burnout**
C **Cast restoration**
D **Amalgam**
E **Enamel**

There are no matches for the terms reparative dentin, dentin, and caries.

FIGURE 7–25

D. **Shovel-shaped incisor syndrome**

FIGURE 7–26

1. E. **All of the above**
2. C. **Secondary hyperparathyroidism** (renal osteodystrophy)

Note: This patient was on dialysis. She may have had renal acidosis, which could in turn have caused the severe erosion.

FIGURE 7–27

A. **Ameloblastoma**

FIGURE 7–28

B. **Sialolith**
D. **Calcified lymph node**

Note: These two can be easily distinguished by performing a sialogram.

FIGURE 7–29

1. C. **Cleft palate**
2. D. **Transposition** (translocation)

FIGURE 7–30

C. **Mandibular torus**

FIGURE 7–31

A **Pulp stone**
B **Tooth-colored filling material**
C **Amalgam restoration**
D **Internal oblique ridge**

There are no matches for the terms external oblique ridge and cast gold restoration.

FIGURE 7–32

D. **The lead apron blocked the beam.**

FIGURE 7–33

A. **Fibrous healing defect.** Note that the canine is clearly missing and that the chronic inflammation could arise from the obvious periodontal disease that is present.

FIGURE 7–34

C. **Buccal exostoses**

FIGURE 7–35

A. **Cleidocranial dysplasia**

Well, how did you do? We hope you enjoyed this and that you had a little bit of fun while you learned!

Index

Note: Page numbers followed by "A" refer to expanded answer discussions.

Abrasion, toothbrush, 62, 70, 145, 170A
Abscess, periapical, 78, 79, 100, 102
Abutment, fixed bridge, tooth as, 87
Acrylic restoration material(s), 47, 48, 52, 73
Adumbration (cervical burn-out), 21, 103, 148, 160A
Air bubble, on film, 32, 163A
Air cells, ethmoid, 15, 16, 17
    anterior, 18
    posterior, 18
  mastoid, 15, 16, 17, 18
Air space, of oropharynx, 15
Air space error, 42, 103, 109, 123, 142
Ala(e), nasal, 107
Alloy partial restoration framework, 53
Alveolar bone, trabecular pattern of, 99, 180A
Alveolar canal, inferior, 11, 12, 14
Alveolar cleft, 107
Amalgam overhang, 80
Amalgam restoration, 47, 48, 52, 54, 148, 152
  retrograde, 83
  with cement base, 59
Amalgam tattoo, 51, 87
  on buccal mucosa, 122
Ameloblastic fibroma, 183A
Ameloblastoma, 104, 150
Amelogenesis imperfecta, 73, 74, 87, 138
Anachoretic pulpitis, sequelae of, 102
Anemia, sickle cell, trabecular pattern of alveolar bone in, 99, 180A
Angle of mandible (gonial angle), 14, 15, 17, 18
Angulation of x-ray beam, and visualization of zygomatic arch, 9, 27, 33, 157A
  horizontal, improper, 21, 22, 29
  vertical, excessive positive, 24, 27, 33, 142, 190A
    inadequate, 22
    inadequate positive, 26

Anhidrotic ectodermal dysplasia, tooth abnormalities in, 82
Ankylosis, 59, 61, 65, 83, 87
Antral mucosa, maxillary, 5
  inflammation of, 112
Apicoectomy, fibrous healing defect after, 116
Apron artifact, 42, 152
Arch, zygomatic, 5, 6, 14, 16, 17
  effect of angulation of x-ray beam on visualization of, 9, 27, 33, 157A
  inferior border of, 8
Artery, lingual, canal of, 13
Articular eminence, 14
Atlantoaxial joint, 16, 17
Atlas, 15
  tubercles of, 15, 123
Attrition, 62, 82, 85, 112, 137
Auditory canal, external, 14, 18
  internal, 18
Autogenous tooth transplant, 60
Automatic processor errors, 28, 162A
Axis, 15
  odontoid process of, 15, 16, 17, 18

B-B pellet image, 134
Bicuspid(s), horizontally positioned, 73
  impacted, 68
  microdont, 73
  supernumerary, 63, 68
  with bulbous root, 80
Bite-block, 51
Bite guide, effect of omission of, 147
Bite-wing tab, 51
Blade implant, 51
Bone(s), alveolar, trabecular pattern of, 99, 180A

Bone(s) (*Continued*)
ethmoid, perpendicular plate of, 18
vomer of, 18
ground glass appearance of, 117
hyoid, 14, 121
ghost image of, 140
loss of, 62, 66
malar, 14, 16
inferior border of, 8
temporal, 6
trauma to, and cyst formation, 95, 178A
Bone marrow defect, of jaw, 99, 180A
Breathing tube, image of, 56
Buccal exostoses, 153
Buccal mucosa, amalgam tattoo on, 122
calcification in, 121, 187A
Buccal object rule, 129–132
Bulimia, 172A
tooth abnormalities in, 71
Bullet fragment image, 122, 187A
B-B pellet causing, localization of, 134
Burn-out, cervical, 21, 103, 148, 160A
Burr tip, 51

Calcification, in buccal mucosa, 121, 187A
of lymph node, 121, 151
of pulp, 62
soft-tissue, 32
Calcium hydroxide pulp cap, 56
Calculus, 54, 62, 73, 90
Canal(s), alveolar, inferior, 11, 12, 14
auditory, external, 14, 18
internal, 18
incisive, 3, 141
cyst of, 109, 141, 190A
superior foramen of, 3, 13, 88
lateral, 68
lingual, 12
as site for lingual artery and vein, 13
mandibular, 10, 11, 12, 14
nutrient, 5, 11, 66, 116
foramen of, 65
prominent-appearing, 82
Caries, 80, 175A
and pulpitis, 81
deep, 62, 76, 77, 78, 103
early, 76, 77
frank, 76, 77
in dentinogenesis imperfecta, 88
incipient, 76, 77
radiation therapy and, 79, 174A
Cast-gold post and core restoration, 48
Cement, 47, 54, 56
Cemental dysplasia (cementoma), 112
periapical, 101, 105, 106, 124, 182A
Cementifying fibroma, 114, 185A
Cementoblastoma, benign, 106, 113, 124,
182A, 184A, 188A
Cementoma (cemental dysplasia), 112
periapical, 101, 105, 106, 124, 182A
Central cementifying fibroma, 114, 185A
Central giant cell granuloma, 123, 147, 188A,
190A
Cervical burn-out, 21, 103, 148, 160A
Cervical vertebra(e), appearance of, as super-
imposed image, due to patient positioning
error, 38

Cervical vertebra(e) (*Continued*)
first, 15
tubercles of, 15, 123
second, 15
odontoid process of, 15, 16, 17, 18
third, 15
Cervical vertebral joint(s), 16, 17
Chemical erosion, of teeth, 71
Cherubism, jaw abnormalities in, 99, 180A
Child(ren), periodontitis in, 110
sequence of tooth eruption in, 49
third molar in, 72
Chrome cobalt restoration, 47
Cingulum, accentuated, 80
Cleft(s), alveolar, 107
palatal, 107, 151
Cleidocranial dysplasia, tooth abnormalities
in, 61, 154
Clinoid process, anterior, 15
posterior, 15
Cloudy sinus, 112, 184A
Complex odontoma, 115, 125, 185A
Composite resin restoration material(s), 47,
54
Compound fracture, of mandible, 103
Compound odontoma, 96, 125, 185A
Condyle, mandibular, 6, 14
head of, 18
depression in, 14
Cone cut, 21, 35
Contaminant, fluoride as, 25
Coronal suture, 15
Coronoid process of mandible, 5, 8, 14, 17, 18
Cortical plate, 5, 12
Cotton roll, 51
effect of omission of, 147
Curving of film, excessive, 24, 161A
Cusp, talon, 68
Cuspid(s), deciduous, retention of, 74
double-rooted, 69
impacted, 74
localization of, 134
Cyst(s), dentigerous, 103, 109, 125
eruptive, 110
incisive canal, 109, 141, 190A
mucous, 86, 102, 115
vs. mucositis, 181A
periapical, 78, 79, 100, 102
periodontal, 97, 140
retention, 86, 102, 115
vs. mucositis, 181A
trauma to bone and, 95, 178A

Deciduous tooth (teeth), absence of, 82
retention of, 74
Delayed eruption, radiation therapy and, 64
Dens evaginatus, 80
Dens in dente, 59, 68, 74, 88
Dental papilla, 138
Dentigerous cyst, 103, 109, 125
Dentin, dysplasia of, 66, 82, 143
sclerotic, 148
secondary, formation of, 59
Dentinogenesis imperfecta, 63, 88
Denture(s), accidental inclusion of, in radio-
graphic examination, 37, 147

Developer solution, artifact(s) produced by, 24, 33, 35, 36, 163A
    effect of different strengths at top and bottom of, 34
    over-warm, and grainy appearance of film, 23, 161A
Diastema, 71, 139
Diffuse sclerosing osteomyelitis, 118
Dilaceration, 72, 86, 100, 137
Dimensional distortion, 26
Dorsum sellae, 15
Double exposure, 28
Double-rooted cuspid, 69
Duct, nasolacrimal, 6

Ear lobe, 14
Ectodermal dysplasia, tooth abnormalities in, 60, 82
Elongation, 26, 161A
Eminence, articular, 14
Emulsion, crimping of, at tooth contacts, 34
    scratching of, 29, 31
Enamel, 148
    hypoplasia of, 70, 73, 82, 172A
Enamel pearl, 61, 82, 85, 90, 130, 137, 176A
    localization of, 130
Enamel pearl artifact, 91, 177A
Endodontic instrument image, 50
Erosion, chemical, of teeth, 71
Eruption of teeth, 86
    delayed, radiation therapy and, 64
    factors compromising, 74
    potential for, 110
    sequence of, 49, 168A
Eruption sequestrum, 111
Eruptive cyst, 110
Ethiodized oil, opacification by, 32
Ethmoid air cells, 15, 16, 17
    anterior, 18
    posterior, 18
Ethmoid bone, perpendicular plate of, 18
    vomer of, 18
Exostosis (exostoses), 116
    buccal, 153
External auditory canal, 14, 18
External oblique ridge, 10, 12, 13, 14
Extraction of tooth, appearance of surrounding sites after, in patient treated for pulpitis, 106
Extrusion, 76
Eyeglass (lens) image, 53

Fibroma, ameloblastic, 183A
    cementifying, 114, 185A
Fibrous dysplasia, 117
Fibrous healing defect, 148, 153
    after apicoectomy, 116
File(s), 50, 52
Filling material, 54, 152
Film(s), adhesion between, in film handling, 22, 160A
    air bubble on, 32, 163A
    bending of corners of, 48, 62, 170A
    contamination of, by fluoride, 25
    dark appearance of, causes of, 29

Film(s) (*Continued*)
    double exposure of, 28
    effect of cassette hang-up on, 43
    effect of light exposure errors on, 41
    effect of premature machine activation on, 43
    excessive curving of, 24, 161A
    fogging of, causes of, 31
    grainy appearance of, over-warm developer solution and, 23, 161A
    light appearance of, causes of, 27
    premature removal of, from fixer solution, 30
    static electricity on, 28, 35
    unsuccessful exposure of, 23, 161A
Film exposure, double, 28
    unsuccessful, 23, 161A
Film handling, adhesion between films in, 22, 160A
    excessive curving of film in, 24, 161A
    finger in, and phalangioma error, 21
Film holder image, 50, 52, 54
Film motion error(s), 23, 30
Film placement, reversed, 30, 162A
Film processing, machine errors in, 28
Finger(s), in film handling, and phalangioma error, 21
Fingernail artifact, 26, 35
Fissure, pterygomaxillary, 14, 15
Fixed bridge, abutment for, tooth as, 87
Fixer solution, artifact(s) produced by, 25, 32, 37
    effect of insufficient quantity of, 34
    effect of premature removal of film from, 30
Floating tooth, 124
Fluoride, as film contaminant, 25
Focal osteoporotic bone marrow defect, of jaw, 99, 180A
Focal sclerosing osteomyelitis, 59, 61, 101
Fogging, causes of, 31
Fold, nasolabial, 4, 98, 148
Foramen (foramina), incisive, 4, 7, 8, 141, 144, 157A
    infraorbital, 17
    jugular, 18
    lingual, 10
    mental, 10, 11, 14, 65, 73, 158A
    of incisive canal, 3, 13, 88
    of nutrient canal, 65
Foramen magnum, 18
Foramen ovale, 18
Foramen spinosum, 18
Forceps (film holder) image, 50, 54
Foreshortening, 24, 25, 70, 172A
Fossa(e), lateral, 7, 139
    mandibular (glenoid), 14
    nasal, 3, 7, 8, 13, 14, 125
        floor of, 16
        lateral wall of, 13, 14, 18, 148
        on submentovertex view of skull, 18
    pituitary, 15
    submandibular, 11
Fracture(s), of incisal edge of incisor, 80
    of mandible, 103
    of root, 89
Frame (eyeglass frame) image, 53
Frontal sinus, 15, 16, 17
Fusion of teeth, 83, 85, 176A

Garré's osteomyelitis, 120
  antibiotics for, 186A
Gauze, 54
Gemination, 86, 145, 176A
Genial tubercle(s), 10
  enlargement of, 108
Ghost images, 14, 140
Giant cell granuloma, 123, 147, 188A, 190A
Glenoid (mandibular) fossa, 14
Gold restoration material, 47, 52–55, 73
Gonial angle (angle of mandible), 14, 15, 17, 18
Grainy film, over-warm developer solution and, 23, 161A
Granuloma(s), giant cell, 123, 147, 188A, 190A
  periapical, 78, 79, 100, 102
Ground glass bone sign, 117
Gutta-percha, 48, 50, 52, 148

Hamular notch, soft-tissue shadow of, 9
Hamulus, 6
Hard palate, 14, 15
  posterior border of, 18
  shadow of, as superimposed image, due to patient positioning error, 40
Hyoid bone, 14, 121
  ghost image of, 140
Hypercementosis, 66, 86, 103
Hyperostosis, 111
  mandibular, 108, 183A
Hyperparathyroidism, secondary, 186A
  tooth abnormalities in, 117, 150, 186A
Hypohidrotic ectodermal dysplasia, tooth abnormalities in, 60

Impacted tooth (teeth), 67, 68, 74, 90
  localization of, 134
Incisive canal, 3, 141
  cyst of, 109, 141, 190A
  superior foramen of, 3, 13, 88
Incisive foramen, 4, 7, 8, 141, 144, 157A
Incisor(s), congenital absence of, 61, 82, 138
  fracture of incisal edge of, 80
  fusion of, 83, 85
  in lingual version, 49
  loss of apical image of, due to patient positioning errors, 38, 39
  microdont, 75
  peg lateral, 75, 107
  restoration of, 112
  rotation of, 66
  shortened roots of, orthodontic treatment and, 144
  shovel-shaped, 149, 185A
  supernumerary, 64
  trauma to, sequelae of, 83, 176A
Infraorbital foramen, 17
Inner table, 15, 16
Innominate line, panoramic, 14
Internal auditory canal, 18
Internal oblique ridge, 11, 12, 13, 152
Inverted Y landmark, 3, 13, 98

Jaw(s), abnormalities of, in cherubism, 99, 180A
  focal osteoporotic bone marrow defect of, 99, 180A
Joint(s), atlantoaxial, 16, 17
  temporomandibular, effect of patient positioning errors on visualization of, 39, 40
Jugular foramen, 18
Juvenile periodontitis, 110

Keratocyst, odontogenic, 120, 182A, 183A, 187A
  dentigerous, 120

Lambdoid suture, 15
Lamina dura, in periodontal disease, 62
  loss of, 103
Lateral canal, 68
Lateral fossa, 7, 139
Lateral view of skull, 15
Lead apron artifact, 152
Leaded glass image, 49
Lens (eyeglass) image, 53
Lentula, 52
Ligament, petroclinoid, 15
Light-exposed film error, 41
Lingual canal, 12
  as site for lingual artery and vein, 13
Lingual foramen, 10
Lingual version, incisor in, 49
Lip(s), lower, line of, 12
  shadow of, 10
  soft tissue of, 13
  soft tissue outline of, 14
  upper, 80
  line of, 7
Localization techniques, 67, 129–134, 144, 146, 171A, 189A
Lymph node(s), calcification of, 121, 151

Machine errors, in film processing, 28
Macrodontia, 81
Magnification, 27, 161A
Malar bone, 14, 16
  inferior border of, 8
Malar process, 9
Mamelons, 69
Mandible, 11, 13, 16, 17
  coronoid process of, 5, 8, 14, 17, 18
  fracture of, 103
  lesions of, benign vs. malignant, 95, 178A
  ramus of, 16, 18
    effect of patient positioning errors on visualization of, 38, 39
    posterior border of, 14, 17
Mandibular anterior occlusal view, 13
Mandibular canal, 10, 11, 12, 14
Mandibular condyle, 6, 14
  head of, 18
    depression in, 14
Mandibular (glenoid) fossa, 14

Mandibular hyperostosis, 108, 183A
Mastoid air cells, 15, 16, 17, 18
Maxilla, zygomatic process of, 8, 9, 14, 15, 18
Maxillary anterior occlusal view, 13
Maxillary antral mucosa, 5
  inflammation of, 112
Maxillary sinus, 3, 8, 14
  anterior wall of, 14
  cloudy appearance of, 112, 184A
  floor of, 5, 14
  inferior border of, 14
  lateral wall of, 18
  medial wall of, 13, 18
  on radiograph(s) of skull, using lateral
    view, 15
    using submentovertex view, 18
    using Waters view, 17
  posterior wall of, 14
  radiopacity associated with, differential di-
    agnosis of, 112
  septum of, 52
Maxillary tuberosity, 8, 14
Meatus, auditory, external, 14, 18
  internal, 18
  nasal, common, 14, 16
    inferior, 16, 148
    middle, 14
Medial sigmoid depression, 8, 14
Median palatal suture, 4
Mental foramen, 10, 11, 14, 65, 73, 158A
Mental ridge, 12, 13
Mesiodens, 67
Metal alloy restoration material(s), 52
Metal object image, 122
  B-B pellet causing, localization of, 134
  eyeglass frames causing, 53
Microdontia, 81
Migration, 142
Molar(s), first, lesions of, 79, 175A
  fourth, eruption of, 86
  impacted, 90
  root tips of, retention of, 97
  second, incomplete apexification of, 79,
    175A
  third, in children, 72
    localization of, 130
  unerupted, 65
Motion error(s), 23, 30, 43
Mucosa, antral, maxillary, 5
  inflammation of, 112
  buccal, amalgam tattoo on, 122
    calcification in, 121, 187A
  periapical, inflammation of, 103
    vs. mucous cyst, 181A
Mucositis, antral, maxillary, 112
  periapical, 103
    vs. mucous cyst, 181A
Mucous cyst, 86, 102, 115
  vs. mucositis, 181A
Mylohyoid line, 11, 12

Nasal fossa, 3, 7, 8, 13, 14, 125
  floor of, 16
  lateral wall of, 13, 14, 18, 148
  on submentovertex view of skull, 18

Nasal septum, 7, 13, 14
  on radiograph(s) of skull, using postero-an-
    terior view, 16
    using Waters view, 17
Nasal spine, anterior, 7, 15, 16
Nasolabial fold, 4, 98, 148
Nasolacrimal duct, 6
Neck chain error, 41
Nose, 4, 5
  ala(e) of, 107
  meatus of, common, 14, 16
    inferior, 16, 148
    middle, 14
  soft tissue of, 14, 148
    outline of, 140
  tip of, 14, 80, 109
Nutrient canal(s), 5, 11, 66, 116
  foramen of, 65
  prominent-appearing, 82

Object magnification rule, 134
Oblique ridge, external, 10, 12, 13, 14
  internal, 11, 12, 13, 152
Occiput, 15
Odontogenic keratocyst, 120, 182A, 183A,
  187A
  dentigerous, 120
Odontoid process of axis, 15, 16, 17, 18
Odontoma, 96, 114, 115, 125, 185A
Oil, opacification by, 32
Open-faced stainless steel crowns, 50
Orbit, 14, 17
  inferior border of, 14
  lateral border of, 16, 17
Orbital plates, cerebral surfaces of, 15
Oropharynx, air space of, 15
Orthodontic band, 53
Orthodontic bracket, 53
Orthodontic tooth movement, 65
Osteogenesis imperfecta, tooth abnormalities
  in, 63, 88
Osteoma, 116
Osteomyelitis, 119
  Garré's, 120
    antibiotics for, 186A
  sclerosing, 59, 61, 101, 118
Osteoporosis, 123, 188A
Osteoporotic bone marrow defect, of jaw, 99,
  180A
Osteosclerosis, 59, 61, 101, 113, 143, 185A
Outer table, 15, 16
Overlapping tooth contacts, cause of appear-
  ance of, 29
Oxygen breathing tube, image of, 56

Paget disease, 118
Palatal suture, median, 4
Palate, cleft, 107, 151
  hard, 14, 15
    posterior border of, 18
    shadow of, as superimposed image, due to
      patient positioning error, 40
  soft, 14

Palatoglossal air space error, 42, 103, 109, 123, 142
Pancentric patient positioning bar, 14
Panoramic innominate line, 14
Panoramic localization, 133–134
Papilla, dental, 138
Paramolar, 64
Patient identification artifact, 33
Patient movement errors, 23, 43, 167A
Patient positioning bar, pancentric, 14
Patient positioning errors, 38–40, 109, 123, 140, 147, 164A–166A, 183A
Periapical abscess, 78, 79, 100, 102
Periapical cemental dysplasia, 101, 105, 106, 124, 182A
Periapical cyst, 78, 79, 100, 102
Periapical granuloma, 78, 79, 100, 102
Periapical mucositis, 103
  vs. mucous cyst, 181A
Pericoronitis, 110, 183A
Perimyolysis, 71
Periodontal cyst, 97, 140
Periodontal disease, and floating tooth, 124
  lamina dura in, 62
Periodontal membrane space, thickening of, 98
Periodontitis, juvenile, 110
Perpendicular plate, of ethmoid bone, 18
Petroclinoid ligament, 15
Petrous ridge, 15, 16
Phalangioma error, from finger in film-handling, 21
Pharynx, posterior wall of, 15
Pin(s), 51
Pin-type implant, 51
Pindborg tumor, 115, 185A
Pituitary fossa, 15
Plate(s), cortical, 5, 12
  orbital, cerebral surfaces of, 15
  perpendicular, of ethmoid bone, 18
  pterygoid, 6
    lateral, 14
Platinum foil, 48
Pliers (film holder) image, 52
Porcelain restoration(s), 47, 48, 51, 51–54, 69
Postero-anterior view of skull, 16
Process(es), clinoid, anterior, 15
    posterior, 15
  coronoid, of mandible, 5, 8, 14, 17, 18
  malar, 9
  odontoid, of axis, 15, 16, 17, 18
  zygomatic, of maxilla, 8, 9, 14, 15, 18
Processing solutions, effect of extreme differences in temperatures of, 34, 163A
Processor errors, 28, 162A
Protective apron artifact, 42, 152
Pterygoid plate, lateral, 14
Pterygoid process, 6
Pterygomaxillary fissure, 14, 15
Pulp, calcification of, 62
  inflammation of. See Pulpitis.
  obliteration of, 65, 75, 112, 173A
  resorption of, 65
Pulp chamber, thistle tube morphology of, 82
Pulp stones, 66, 139, 152
Pulpitis, 85, 176A, 181A
  anachoretic, sequelae of, 102
  caries and, 81

Pulpitis (Continued)
  extraction of tooth for, appearance of surrounding sites after, 106, 182A

Radiation caries, 79, 174A
Radiation stunting, 64
Ramus of mandible, 16, 18
  effect of patient positioning errors on visualization of, 38, 39
  posterior border of, 14, 17
Resin restoration material(s), 54
Resorption, 69
  of pulp, 65
  of roots, 59, 83
Restoration material(s), 47, 48, 50–56, 112, 148, 152
Retention cyst, 86, 102, 115
  vs. mucositis, 181A
Retentive pin, 51
Reticulation, 34, 163A
Reversed film placement, 30, 162A
Reversed smile line, due to patient positioning error, 40
Ridge, mental, 12, 13
  oblique, external, 10, 12, 13, 14
    internal, 11, 12, 13, 152
  petrous, 15, 16
  supraorbital, 16, 17
Rieger's syndrome, 170A
  tooth abnormalities in, 61
Roller error, 28, 162A
Root(s), bulbous, of bicuspid, 80
  double, cuspid, 69
  fracture of, 89
  incisor, shortened, orthodontic treatment and, 144
  resorption of, 59, 83
  supernumerary, 62, 66, 81, 87, 131
    localization of, 131
  tapered, 62
Root canal space, obliteration of, 59, 103
Root tips, retention of, 97, 98, 179A
Rotation, of incisor, 66
Rubber, 51
Rubber dam frame image, 50

Salivary gland depression, 96, 108, 144, 178A, 182A
Same-on-lingual-opposite-on-buccal rule, 133–134
Schizodontism, 86, 145, 176A
Sclerosing osteomyelitis, 59, 61, 101, 118
Sclerosis, dentinal, 148
  socket, 100, 141
Scratching, of emulsion, 29, 31
Septum (septa), maxillary sinus, 52
  nasal, 7, 13, 14
    on radiograph(s) of skull, using postero-anterior view, 16
    using Waters view, 17
Sequestrum, eruption, 111
Shotgun pellet image, 32
Shoulder strap artifact, 42, 167A
Shovel-shaped incisor syndrome, 149, 185A

Sialolith, 98, 151, 179A
Sickle cell anemia, trabecular pattern of al-
    veolar bone in, 99, 180A
Sigmoid depression, 8, 14
Sigmoid notch, 14
Silicate restoration, 47
Silicophosphate cement restoration, 47
Silver alloy restoration, 48, 50
    localization of, 131, 132
Silver points, 52
Sinus(es), frontal, 15, 16, 17
    maxillary, 3, 8, 14
        anterior wall of, 14
        cloudy appearance of, 112, 184A
        floor of, 5, 14
        inferior border of, 14
        lateral wall of, 18
        medial wall of, 13, 18
        on radiograph(s) of skull, using lateral
            view, 15
            using submentovertex view, 18
            using Waters view, 17
        posterior wall of, 14
        radiopacity associated with, differential
            diagnosis of, 112
        septum of, 52
    sphenoid, 15, 16, 17, 18
Sinus recess, 4, 142
Skull, lateral view of, 15
    postero-anterior view of, 16
    submentovertex view of, 18
    Waters view of, 17
Smile line, effect of patient positioning errors
    on visualization of, 39, 40
Socket sclerosis, 100, 141
Soft palate, 14
Soft-tissue calcification, 32
Sphenoid sinus, 15, 16, 17, 18
Spine, nasal, anterior, 7, 15, 16
Stainless steel crown, 50, 55
Stainless steel wire splint, 49
Static electricity, on film, 28, 35
Stomach acid, effect of, on teeth, 71
Stunting of teeth, radiation therapy and, 64
Submandibular fossa, 11
Submentovertex view of skull, 18
Submerged tooth, 59, 62, 170A
Supernumerary root(s), 62, 66, 81, 87, 131
    localization of, 131
Supernumerary tooth (teeth), 63, 64, 68
Supraeruption, 76
Supraorbital ridge, 16, 17
Suture(s), coronal, 15
    lambdoid, 15
    palatal, median, 4
Suture needle image, 54
Synodontism, 83, 85, 176A

Talon cusp, 68
Taurodontism, 63
Teeth. See *Tooth.*
Temporal bone, 6
Temporomandibular joint, effect of patient po-
    sitioning errors on visualization of, 39, 40
Thistle tube pulp chamber, 82

Tongue, 12, 13, 15
    shadow of, 138
Tooth (teeth), abnormalities of, in anhidrotic
        ectodermal dysplasia, 82
    in bulimia, 71
    in cleidocranial dysplasia, 61, 154
    in hypohidrotic ectodermal dysplasia, 60
    in osteogenesis imperfecta, 63, 88
    in Rieger's syndrome, 61
    in secondary hyperparathyroidism, 117,
        150, 186A
    size-related, 81
    as abutment for fixed bridge, 87
    autogenous transplant of, 60
    chemical erosion of, 71
    condition of, age factors in, 49
    congenital absence of, 61, 82, 138
    deciduous, absence of, 82
        retention of, 74
    distal drift of, 72
    effect of patient positioning errors on visu-
        alization of, 38–40, 164A–166A
    effect of stomach acid on, 71
    eruption of, 86
        delayed, radiation therapy and, 64
        factors compromising, 74
        potential for, 110
        sequence of, 49, 168A
    extraction of, appearance of surrounding
        sites after, in patient treated for pulpitis,
        106
    floating, 124
    fusion of, 83, 85, 176A
    impacted, 67, 68, 74, 90
        localization of, 134
    loss of apical image of, due to patient posi-
        tioning errors, 38, 39, 40
    orthodontic movement of, 65
    stunting of, radiation therapy and, 64
    submerged, 59, 62, 170A
    supernumerary, 63, 64, 68
    transplant of, autogenous, 60
    transposition (translocation) of, 67, 151
    trauma to, 49, 83
        sequelae of, 84, 176A
    unerupted, 65
Tooth contacts, crimping of emulsion at, 34
    overlapping appearance of, cause of, 29
Toothbrush abrasion, 62, 70, 145, 170A
Torus (tori), 68, 97, 111, 112, 184A
Translocation (transposition), 67, 151
Transplant of tooth, autogenous, 60
Transposition (translocation), 67, 151
Trauma, to bone, and cyst formation, 95,
        178A
    to teeth, 49, 83
        sequelae of, 84, 176A
Tubercle(s), genial, 10
        enlargement of, 108
    of atlas, 15, 123
Tuberosity, maxillary, 8, 14
Tubing, oxygen, image of, 56
Tumor, Pindborg, 115, 185A
Turbinate(s), inferior, 7, 16, 148

Unerupted tooth, 65

Vein, lingual, canal of, 13
Vertebra(e), appearance of, as superimposed
    image, due to patient positioning errors,
    38, 40
  C-1, 15
    tubercles of, 15, 123
  C-2, 15
    odontoid process of, 15, 16, 17, 18
  C-3, 15
Vertebral joint(s), C-1–C-2, 16, 17
Vomer, of ethmoid bone, 18
Vomiting, and chemical erosion of teeth, 71

Waters view of skull, 17
Wire restoration material, 51, 52, 53

X-ray beam, angulation of, and visualization
    of zygomatic arch, 9, 27, 33, 157A

X-ray beam (*Continued*)
    angulation of, horizontal, improper, 21, 22,
      29
    vertical, excessive positive, 24, 27, 33,
      142, 190A
    inadequate, 22
    inadequate positive, 26
X-ray machine, as source of motion error, 23

Y landmark, inverted, 3, 13, 98

Zinc oxide–eugenol cement, 55
Zygomatic arch, 5, 6, 14, 16, 17
    effect of angulation of x-ray beam on visu-
      alization of, 9, 27, 33, 157A
    inferior border of, 8
Zygomatic process of maxilla, 8, 9, 14, 15, 18